What Others Are Saying...

"If you're thinking of cosmetic surgery or just want to learn more, this is the book. Dr. Kotler, one of the top cosmetic surgeons in the United States, guides you through the procedures and what each entails—from costs to recovery times. You will truly be informed..."
-Mary Ann Malloy, MD
Women's health expert, NBC

"Cosmetic surgery can be a life-changing decision, and Dr. Kotler relays valuable information so the public can make an informed decision. An excellent resource for both doctor and patient. Sound decisions translate to peace of mind—an important factor when considering plastic surgery."
-Howard Murad, MD
Assistant Clinical Professor of Dermatology, UCLA

"The secrets of finding a cosmetic surgeon who is right for you. A must have book for anyone contemplating this type of surgery."
-Dr. Earl Mindell
Author, *Vitamin, Herb* and *Diet Bibles*

"Dr. Robert Kotler, an acknowledged master of facial plastic surgery has written an informative, easy, well-organized and humorous 'must read' for the patient who requires education regarding cosmetic surgery in order to be well versed in all nuances and protected from the pitfalls."
-Jeremy L. Freeman, MD
Professor of Otolaryngology, University of Toronto

"A bible for the consumer who is looking for rejuvenation, and is concerned about what procedure they really need and who's the best to do it. Contains checklists to make sure they stay on the right track."
-James E. Fulton Jr., MD, PhD, Co-Developer Retin-A®

"A thorough consumer's guide highlighting all important areas one should consider when contemplating cosmetic surgery. Consumers should do their homework, and this book is invaluable toward that end."
-David B. Barinholtz, MD, Clinical Associate
University of Chicago, Pritzker School of Medicine

"Complete and concise. In today's complex cosmetic surgery world, there are more choices for procedures, operating facilities and surgeons. That's why the consumer needs this book."
-Kurt J. Wagner, MD, FACS
Board certified plastic surgeon and author

"This book should be the starting point for anyone even day-dreaming of cosmetic surgery. Eminently readable, engrossing, informative it provides a simply-told education in what these magical and mysterious procedures are, how they work, what can realistically go wrong, and how to prevent it. Dr. Kotler writes conversationally, like a friend who cares, but a friend who is also one of the foremost experts in this technical yet artistic business. He dares to be honest about the whole process."

-Barbara Sternig
Journalist and author

"In language every patient can understand, Dr. Kotler entwines humor with common sense, intelligent decision making based on informed facts, and addresses issues to consider when planning cosmetic surgery. He leads you step by step through the discovery, performance, and recovery periods ... and he leaves you smiling."

-Maggie Lockridge, RN
Administrator, Shanteque, A Recovery Retreat

"In this era when patients are becoming more involved in their medical care, Dr. Kotler's book is certainly timely. It is a tremendous resource for patients contemplating cosmetic and/or reconstructive surgery."

-Paul Lambert, MD
Professor, Otolaryngology-Head and Neck Surgery
Medical University of South Carolina

"Contains valuable information that will be of great interest to patients who are considering cosmetic surgery, particularly choosing a surgeon on the basis of training, experience, and expertise."

-John W. Shore, MD, FACS
President, American Society of Ophthalmic
Plastic and Reconstructive Surgery

"... distills decades of clinical experience into a seasoned view of the cosmetic surgery landscape, where Dr. Kotler guides the patient through the labyrinth of choices and potential obstacles with the same warm and generous sense of caring that has made him an outstanding success in his field. Recommended for the reader who is contemplating elective cosmetic surgery."

-Richard G. Glogau, MD
Professor of Dermatology, University of California

"The book is a gem! It provides essential, timely advice on the strengths and pitfalls of cosmetic surgery. If you are considering optimizing your ppearance with any cosmetic surgical and non-surgical procedure, Secrets of a Beverly Hills Cosmetic Surgeon *is a must read!"*

-Rosalene Glickman, Ph.D
President, The World Academy of Personal Development

SECRETS OF A BEVERLY HILLS COSMETIC SURGEON

The Expert's Guide to Safe, Successful Surgery

Robert Kotler, MD, FACS

*A defective soul cannot be corrected on the face, but a defect on the face, if you correct it, **can** correct the soul.*
                                        -Jacques Cousteau

SECRETS OF A BEVERLY HILLS COSMETIC SURGEON
Robert Kotler, MD, FACS

Published by:
Ernest Mitchell Publishers
P.O. Box 15371
Beverly Hills, CA 90209-1371
Phone: 1-888-599-3400
Info at www.surgerysecrets.com

Printed in the United States of America
10 9 8 7 6 5 4 3 2 1

Library of Congress Control Number: 2001 126802
ISBN: 0-9712262-0-2 (Hardbound)

Disclaimer

This book is designed to provide information about the subject matter covered.

It is not the purpose of this book to reprint all the information that is otherwise available to the author and/or publisher, but to complement, amplify and supplement. You are urged to read all available material.

Every effort has been made to make this book as complete and as accurate as possible. However, there may be mistakes both typographical and in content. Therefore, this text should be used only as a general guide.

The purpose of this book is to educate. The author and Ernest Mitchell Publishers shall have neither liability nor responsibility to any person or entity with respect to any loss or damage caused, directly or indirectly by the information contained in this book.

Text Design: Carolyn Porter, One-On-One Book Production
Cover Design: Peter Thorpe and One-On-One Book Production

Cartoons on pages 133 and 154 are used with permission of the Cartoon Bank © 2002 *The New Yorker* Collection from cartoonbank.com All rights reserved. Cartoon on page 181— MISTER BUFFO © 1996 Joe Martin. Dist. By UNIVERSAL PRESS SYNDICATE. Reprinted with permission . All rights reserved. Cartoon on page 198—BIZARRO © 2001 by Dan Piraro. Reprinted with permission of UNIVERSAL PRESS SYNDICATE. All rights reserved.

DEDICATION

To my parents, my family, my teachers and Neil Baum, MD.

In memory of my brother Ed Kotler (1947-1999), and my lifelong friend Jay Shapiro (1942-2000), the bravest people I have ever known. Author royalties will benefit the Ed Kotler Chapter of the Leukemia Research Foundation, Evanston, Il.

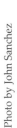

ABOUT THE AUTHOR

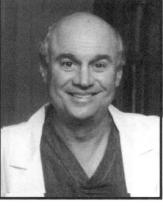

Robert Kotler, MD, FACS

Robert Kotler, MD, FACS, practices cosmetic facial surgery, exclusively, in Beverly Hills, California.

Born in Chicago, Dr. Kotler attended the University of Wisconsin and is a graduate of Northwestern University Medical School. He served his general surgery residency at Cook County Hospital in Chicago. His specialty residency training in surgery of the face, head and neck was served at Cook County Hospital, Northwestern University Hospitals, and the University of Illinois Hospitals. Dr. Kotler is board certified, by the American Board of Otolaryngology/Head and Neck Surgery.

Major Kotler was Chief of Head and Neck Surgery at the DeWitt Army Hospital, Fort Belvoir, Virginia, and a consultant and residency program instructor at the Walter Reed Army Medical Center, Washington, D.C., during his service in the U.S. Army Medical Corps.

Following military service, Dr. Kotler served a fellowship in cosmetic facial surgery in Los Angeles, sponsored by the American Academy of Facial Plastic and Reconstructive Surgery.

Dr. Kotler is the founder of the Cosmetic Surgery Specialists Medical Group of Beverly Hills. In addition to his private practice, he is a Clinical Instructor in the Division of Head and Neck Surgery, Department of Surgery, UCLA Center for the Health Sciences. He is a Consultant and Attending Surgeon at the Veterans' Medical Center, West Los Angeles. Dr. Kotler has served as a Commissioner and Regional Consultant to the Medical Board of California, and as a Medical Consultant to the City and County of Los Angeles.

Dr. Kotler is the author of *The Consumer's Guidebook To Cosmetic Facial Surgery,* a consumer-oriented guidebook. He also wrote the medical text, *Chemical Rejuvenation of the Face,* used by physicians worldwide. Dr. Kotler is credited with 51 medical publications and presentations and he has been a contributor to 12 medical textbooks and books for the public.

As a spokesperson for cosmetic surgeons, Dr. Kotler has been a guest on numerous local and national radio and television programs including *Oprah, CBS News, 48 Hours, CNN, Fox News* and has been interviewed by *Time, Self, McCalls, Men's Health, Allure, Men's Fitness, Los Angeles Magazine, W, Woman's Day, The Chicago Sun-Times, Los Angeles Times, Detroit Press, Arizona Republic, Denver Post, Cincinnati Enquirer, Parade, USA Today* and the *National Enquirer.*

TABLE OF CONTENTS

Teachers and Books are the Springs from which the Waters of Knowledge Flow.
    – Inscription on the Plaza Fountain, Memorial Library,
University of Wisconsin, Madison

Acknowledgments

...WITH APPRECIATION...

The road to becoming a master cosmetic surgeon is long, arduous and challenging. Without inspiring teachers and mentors, supportive colleagues and associates and attentive and dedicated staff, the journey is uncomfortable and uncertain.

Appreciation—in large doses—is due the faculty, at the University of Illinois Medical Center's Department of Head and Neck Surgery in Chicago.

I particularly want to thank Illinois' M. Eugene Tardy, Jr., MD, an extraordinarily gifted surgeon, demanding teacher and prolific author. In addition to imparting and transplanting fundamental principles of tissue management, as well as the nuances of cosmetic—particularly nasal—surgery, Dr. Tardy inspired my interest in medical photography. He encouraged me to study under Helen Silver who was the Chief Medical Photographer at the University of Illinois Eye and Ear Infirmary. That training in photography led to the creation of my first medical textbook, *Chemical Rejuvenation of the Face.* Drs. Paul Holinger, Albert Andrews, Jr., Richard Buckingham, and Francis Lederer, authors of the unique and magnificent *The Atlas of Otorhinolaryngology and Bronchosophagology,* further stimulated my interest in capturing medical "photo opportunities," and then using these as a vehicle for superior teaching—so critical in our visual specialty.

Morrison Beers, MD, an early giant in Chicago cosmetic surgery, brought to our department the knowledge, skills and perspective of our brethren in plastic surgery, and was extremely generous with his time for this young surgeon. Dr. Beers was particularly inspiring because he was one of the pioneer cosmetic surgeons of his era, having the foresight to pursue additional training as a fellow in cosmetic surgery following his residency. Witnessing his superior talent, I saw the value of that additional, highly-focused training known as fellowship.

In California, following residency, board certification, and military service, I served that fellowship—the postgraduate apprenticeship that represents a young cosmetic surgeon's "finishing school"—under the late Morey Parkes, MD, a major figure in the first "class" of pioneers in facial cosmetic surgery—a newly emerging superspecialty. From Dr. Parkes and his associate, Frank Kamer, MD, I learned the art as well as the science of cosmetic facial surgery. Dr. Parkes was a "master surgeon"—the highest accolade surgeons bestow upon a colleague. Still greatly valued is that fellowship experience.

If I have been able to see farther, it was because I stood on the shoulders of giants.

-Sir Isaac Newton

My interest in chemical skin peeling (nonsurgical facial rejuvenation) was inspired and nurtured by Richard Ariagno, MD, of Northwestern University Medical School in Chicago. I owe deep gratitude to him for generously sharing his long experience with this splendid and miraculous process, which will be described and illustrated later in this book.

Through serendipity, my first practice association was an association with one of Dr. Ariagno's star disciples, Jack P. Startz, MD, of Beverly Hills. Dr. Startz, a pharmacist as well as facial surgeon, built upon his work under Dr. Ariagno to become one of the world's pre-eminent chemical face peelers. From Dr. Startz, I was able to enhance my abilities in all areas of facial cosmetic surgery— particularly the chemical peeling procedure. This procedure has been a source of pride and satisfaction throughout my career. As a junior associate of Dr. Startz, I served what was effectively a second cosmetic surgery fellowship. This fortuitously provided yet another "finishing school" opportunity.

During my Army service, on leave in New York City, I had a "surgical epiphany." As a visitor to Howard Diamond, MD's operating room, I witnessed technical expertise and unusual efficiency that far surpassed the norm. He was the world's most prolific nasal surgeon with over 15,000 nasal surgeries performed in his career, and with Dr. Diamond, my education did not end with "the last stitch." He is a man of varied interests and talents: a rollicking pianist, a collector of art and antiques, and a first-class raconteur. And yet, despite his unparalleled accomplishments and superior talents and attributes, he is unusually unpretentious. By sharing with me his philosophies, strategies, methods and peerless operative techniques, I was able to enhance my abilities and hence have received special satisfaction performing nasal surgery. And since nasal cosmetic surgery is unquestionably the most challenging and complicated of all cosmetic surgeries, I greatly value Dr. Diamond's tutelage. How lucky I was to have discovered him. Among giants, he stands the tallest.

No Man is an Island.

– John Donne

Unbounded appreciation goes to my devoted and extraordinarily skillful surgical assistant, Tae Yeun Lee. She lends quiet efficiency and competency, in addition to extraordinary reliability to our surgical services. My work isn't work when Mrs. Lee is assisting. It's been that way for over 17 years.

My office staff—Mary Jakubowitz, Karel Rall, Margie Falk, Jennifer Ginsburg—critiqued and provided technical support for the production of this book, while keeping the office sailing on a smooth course.

The manuscript was transcribed by Sandalwood Transcription Service. Day or night, weekday or weekend, they always "got it done."

During the manuscript preparation, Shannon Melamed word-processed countless edits and somehow found time to complete high school and begin college.

Natalie Eslamboli, Shannon's sidekick, ably assisted in cataloguing quotations and references.

Consultation, word processing and general support from Helaine, Lauren and Lindsey Kotler (In London, Ann Arbor and Los Angeles. Thank heaven for laptops and e-mail!) Review by Wendy Taylor, English teacher Elizabeth Guillen, all-around communication-maven Gary Slayman and cosmetic surgery's most vocal champion, Robert Griffith.

Technical and special editing by "Joanna and Isabel." Joanna Frichtel, BSN, RN, Patient Advisor and Skin Care Specialist at our Cosmetic Surgery Specialists Medical Group of Beverly Hills for her valued input to Appendix A, Nonsurgical Techniques, Office Procedures, and Anti-Aging Skin Care Products. From Texas, concept development and special editing by Isabel Stoltzman. A top co-pilot. If the book reads easily and keeps your attention, thank Isabel; she knows how to turn a phrase.

Barbara Lehman, of Charlotte, North Carolina brainstormed cover concept and design and brutally enforced her rigid code of word economy. A blessing to the author, once crowned the "King of Run-On Sentences."

Keith Wahl, MD FACS, of La Jolla, California, one of our most innovative and talented colleagues—as both surgeon and artist—reviewed the manuscript. His input was golden.

Young Kim, MD, Ph.D., resident surgeon in the Division of Head and Neck Surgery, at UCLA. Dr. Kim, who also earned a Ph.D. while in medical school, has completed three of the six years of our program's prescribed training. He reviewed Chapters 2, 3, and 4 which discuss today's post-graduate medical education for aspiring cosmetic surgeons. His critique of this portion of the book was valuable: he is living daily that very post-graduate life. Only those aboard the ship can understand the voyage.

The author appreciates the thoughtful and practical recommendations and observations submitted by the following peer reviewers and writers who gave so generously of their time: Howard Murad, MD, Lillian Glass, PhD, Earl Mindell, RPh, PhD, Stephen H. Mandy, MD, David Barinholtz, MD, Mary Ann Malloy, MD, Gerald S. Berke, MD, Kurt J. Wagner, MD, John W. Shore, MD, Jeremy L. Freeman, MD, James E. Fulton Jr., MD, PhD, Richard Goode, MD, Athleo L. Cambre, MD, L. Leslie Bolton, MD, Bob Simons, MD, Mike Liponi, Shan Baker, MD, Maggie Lockridge, RN, Barry Glazer, MD, Richard Trubo, Wendy Borrow-Johnson, Barbara Glass, Michael Levine, Anita Talbert, Barbara Sternig and Eleni-Dayle Iversen.

Kotler, Sacher tells me you're going to Chicago next year to start medical school. You're going to be a doctor, huh? Remind me never to get sick.

-Ernest Mitchell
Madison, WI
December 1962

To the consultants at Ernest Mitchell Publishers, a deep bow. During the 1960s Ernie's "Brothers" were clever writers and publishers of a gossipy, semi-underground newsletter *The Omegan* that was the University of Wisconsin's equivalent of today's *National Enquirer.*

40 years later, Ernie's disciples—some of whom are accomplished scriptwriters, producers and published authors—answered this author's call to once again consult, review, and edit, edit, edit.

Photo Editors for facial surgery photographs: Gene Coffman, Lawrence Joseph Gardner, Mlodinoff. For body photos: John Hoffman. Medical Consultants: James (author of *Save Your Knees*) Fox, MD, Skip Holden, MD. Researchers: Stuart Horowitz, Michael O.X. Kesselman, Jerry Berliant. History Consultants: Saul O.Wexler, Mike (co-author of *Che Guevera and the FBI*) Smith, Paul Wolff, Milt Greenblatt, Ron Futterman. Joke selection: Mike Davis, MD, Kenny Pearl, A. Norman Enright, Dick Rovnick, Phil Fidler, Jim (producer of *Airplane, Naked Gun* series) Abraham. Cartoon selection: "The Golds," Marshall Hobbs. Dental Consultants: Robert "No Novocain" Lubar, DDS; Gil Stein, DDS. Fact checkers: Stu Maltz, Mark Alper, BS, RPh.

Deep gratitude for their input, suggestions, and critiquing services: Joel and Susan, Diane and Richard, Lou and Tina, Allen and Marlene, Maureen, B.J., Dana, Lee and Marley Kotler, Zaps and Ila, Marcia Myerberg, Elliot & Marilyn, Bob and Ileene, Bill and Sue, Hal and Sandy, Suzie, and to Nancy Randolf Greenway.

Special mention to: Arlene Bronstein and Chuck and Nancy Cooper of Chicago for their merciless editing and wise advice. David Knowles and Carl Turner for relentlessly sharpening the author's focus and mission.

Very Special Thanks To...

… Dan Poynter. If you are not a full-time author, I do not know how you write a book without this man's help. Bought his books, took his course, devoured his special online newsletter, and I was on my way. He simplifies and creates the roadmap for what is quite a daunting task. If you are a rookie writer, before you pick up a pen, pick up Dan's books. And then pick up the phone and speak with him.

…Carolyn Porter and Alan Gadney of One-On-One Book Production and Marketing. When I first embarked on this writing task, I had not heard the phrase "Book Shepherd." Carolyn and Alan were my shepherds. They made it happen; they smoothly transformed this author's words into a book and then helped deliver it to you, the reader. Real pros, with encyclopedic knowledge of the book publishing and distribution world. On-time, on-target. Their enthusiasm is contagious; how great to work with them.

…Cheryl Spring. A valued consultant and no-holds-barred critic for nearly 20 years. Always a fountain of common sense. Stole time from her retirement and golf games to lend a most appreciated hand.

…Barbara R.E. Glass. Writer and NBC 5 commentator; Chicago's #1 fashion maven. Owns that special sense of style not seen since Mary Gage Peterson. Cherished friend for over 50 years.

…Irwin Zucker, founder, backbone and guiding light, as well as comedian-in-residence, of the Book Publicists of Southern California. Most importantly, Irwin is a man of unusual generosity, consideration and devotion who kept the flame of my book-writing interest burning for years. And, thankfully, Irwin makes it all fun.

…Melvin Powers. Hit songwriter. Successful advertising man. Breeder of horses. Mail order and marketing legend. Book publisher to all the world, in several languages. And, perhaps most significantly, on Sundays, Irwin Zucker's loyal tennis partner. Melvin was my book-writing mentor and resident mind expander. It just could not have happened without him—he hooked me on authorship ten years ago and was the inspiration for my first book for the public, *The Consumer's Guidebook To Cosmetic Facial Surgery.*

…Earl Mindell, RPh, PhD, I have had the good fortune to know Dr. Earl Mindell for many years. Earl is one of the medical world's great educational resources with 45 books written about vitamins and nutrition, an important area somehow overlooked by many medical doctors. Earl Mindell's *Vitamin Bible,* alone, has sold 10 million copies worldwide. A special treat for me, when receiving Earl's input, was that we met at his home office, a detached stunning mock-up of an old-time pharmacy, complete with 100 year old prescription blanks and jars of medicinals long ago forgotten by the medical profession. As one who worked part-time in a somewhat similar "drug store," during high school, meeting with Earl was a strong dose of nostalgia.

...Jay Abraham. Author, consultant, strategist, and unique mind expander. How fortunate to know him, to be his pupil and to enjoy him. An American original. Always challenging our thinking. Jay exemplifies the title of his recent best-selling book, *Getting Everything You Can Out of All You've Got.* He sure does it, and he helps students like yours truly do the same. Our 28-minute video—*About Face*— was Jay's brainchild and quite a kid it was; we were flooded with requests when it premiered. And it is still popular and regarded as the standard of educational excellence for our specialty.

...Rennie Gabriel. Author, publisher, "coach," stimulator (a new title!), motorcyclist. He sees beyond the average field of vision. A concept multiplier. After meeting with Rennie, your mind is racing as fast as a new Harley!

...Diana Rosen. Author, editor, writing consultant. Dry humorist. Always asked me provocative questions that made this a better book for you. Diana's latest book, American Pride, (Citadel) is a nifty, post-September 11 reminder of our country's greatness. A good read.

...Arnold Klein, MD, recognized by our specialty as the "world champion" of Collagen® injections, reviewed Appendix A's section on filling materials. I appreciated and valued Arnie's input because no doctor has more experience nor has ever better summarized for us the current state-of-the-art of filling materials. In fact, the classic medical paper on the subject, written by Dr. Klein and Dr. Melvin Elson, that appeared in the journal *Dermatologic Surgery* was honored by the journal's editors as the "Millennium Paper".

Share Your Knowledge!
– Francis Lederer, MD

That above order was given to me, and to those who came before me, by the late Francis Lederer, M.D., Professor of Head and Neck Surgery, at the giant University of Illinois Medical Center in Chicago. "The Chief," one of the renowned pioneers and world figures of our specialty, served as Department Chairman for over thirty years – at "a dollar a year". He loved his work. Dr. Lederer, also a Navy Captain and Consultant to the Surgeon General, wrote the last major, single-author textbook of head and neck surgery, had a captivating, sparkle-in-the-eye personality, loved teaching, and imparted a taste for it to me and his other trainees and medical students. Our warm memory of Professor Lederer lives on and so does his teaching program, stronger than ever. That residency has trained more specialists and subspecialists in surgery of the head and neck than any other. And, "The Chief's" admonition, to Share Your Knowledge!, helped drive many of us to become teachers and writers.

Since the ability to carry one's message to colleagues, to students, to patients, and to the public requires an additional set of communicative skills, I acknowledge these masters who stimulated, nurtured and refined my speaking and writing talents, whatever they may be.

My "basic training" in expository writing was conducted by Von Steuben High School English teacher extraordinaire, Burl Covan. He got me started. And there was probably some subliminal influence from my father, A.B. Kotler, a newspaper sportswriter when at Chicago's Harrison High. My dad has always had a way with words. His Letters to the Editor to the Chicago newspapers are gems. Years later, my friends remind me, with a chuckle, of having read my father's written apology for having publicly supported a presidential candidate who became a rather disappointing chief executive.

Public speaking has never been a burden. For that, thank yous are in order to University of Wisconsin Speech Professor John Wilson; Dale Carnegie, Larry "Killer" Keller and Nick Bizzio.

Here in Los Angeles, Anne Ready, of the eponymous *Ready for Media*, honed my capabilities as a talk show guest. Thanks to her, it was and still is fun. And when Regis called, and later Oprah, I was indeed "ready for media." Harry Feurer, Robert Rosell, and Andrew and Esther Schorr trained me to succinctly and clearly present often complex technical information to the public. They prepared me for our now quite famous, 28-minute video, *About Face.* There are none better than these folks, believe me.

My continuing education in the art of communication is provided by these world class authors, teachers, and lecturers, many of whom have become valued, personal friends: Allen Bernstein, Jerry Fisher, Seth Godin, Gary Halbert, Dan Kennedy, Conrad Levinson, Lyn Sahr, Yanik Silver, Joe Sugarman and Dottie Walters. I read and reread their books, listened to their audiotapes, watched their videos, and attended their seminars. If indeed *Teachers and Books are the Springs from which the Waters of Knowledge Flow,* I've had a great chance to ride on a torrent of talent. Thank you ladies and gentlemen. I so greatly respect your creativity and your lofty achievements.

Finally, but very importantly, without the graciousness of my patients, whose before and after photos and letters they allowed me to share with you, this book could not be meaningful. Thank you, my friends.

AUTHOR'S INTRODUCTION

No Gossip Here...

This is not an exposé of which Hollywood star had a facelift. No, the *National Enquirer, Globe* and *Star* specialize in that. And, I must admit, they are very good at it, despite our strenuous efforts to protect the privacy of all our patients – including celebrities.

This book runs a bit deeper. Its aim is to teach you, so that wherever you live, you, too, can have the same top-quality cosmetic surgery that most (obviously not all) performers and celebrities have. It is a serious, no-fluff guidebook: not a gossip column. Yes, it takes you behind the scenes, not to the dressing room, but to the doctors' offices and their operating rooms. You will learn the internal workings of this glamorous—but poorly understood—young, medical specialty.

You Need Insider Information

This book is a must; choosing a cosmetic surgeon is not simple. When it comes to your appearance, you want to be sure. You do not want to have regrets. You want to do it right the first time.

My role is to teach you to discriminate between superior and substandard results and recognize the credentials and qualifications of the most skilled practitioners. Anyone considering cosmetic surgery should know what to expect from a consultation, and be armed with specific questions about anesthesia, fees, and even whether or not the surgeon does all or just part of the operation.

Defining Cosmetic Surgery

What is the difference between **plastic surgery** and **cosmetic surgery?**

Some mistakenly use the terms plastic surgery and cosmetic surgery interchangeably. They do not mean the same thing; they are not synonymous.

Plastic surgery describes any surgery, on any part of the body that changes form and/or function. The root word, plas, from Greek, means "to form or shape."

Plastic surgery is a two-component specialty: reconstructive surgery and cosmetic surgery. Reconstructive surgery seeks to restore appearance and function to a pre-injury or pre-tumor state. Here are some of the more common reconstructive procedures: skin grafting for burns, covering bed sores with natural tissue, correcting congenital deformities, management of burns, repairing injuries, limb transplantation, tumor removal and tissue reconstruction.

Reconstructive plastic surgery has been performed for hundreds of years; some rudimentary repair procedures were done thousands of years ago during the time of Hippocrates (460-370 BC).

Cosmetic surgery is a much more limited category of plastic surgery. Cosmetic procedures aim to surpass nature by improving our natural appearance or by reversing the signs of aging. Facelifting, breast augmentation, wrinkle removal, and nasal cosmetic surgery are among the procedures performed daily that either make us look better and/or younger.

The first documented cosmetic surgical procedures upon the face, for example, were performed late in the nineteenth century. But most of the long strides in cosmetic surgery have occurred only in the last 40 years.

Now you understand that all cosmetic surgery is plastic surgery, but not all plastic surgery is cosmetic.

THE FAMILY TREE OF PLASTIC SURGERY

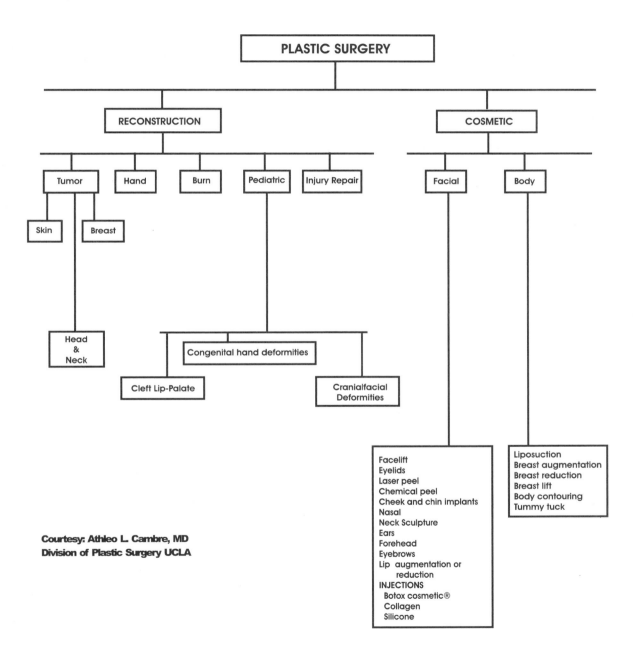

Courtesy: Athleo L. Cambre, MD
Division of Plastic Surgery UCLA

Program Notes

Before we start, a couple of program notes. I cannot cover all details and technicalities of all the procedures within the realm of cosmetic surgery. My scope is limited to the thirteen most common, effective, well-established core procedures. The important ones that make big differences. **Appendix B** lists them in a spreadsheet format for an at-a-glance review. **Appendix A** lists lesser procedures and minor skin treatments.

Patient comments, interspersed throughout the text, are quoted verbatim from written notes and letters received by us. To protect patient confidentiality, complete identification is not provided.

Finally, in referring to doctors, patients and others, I shall use "he." This is not to imply that there are not female doctors; of course there are. Because it is somewhat cumbersome to constantly use "he or she," as a matter of routine, the masculine gender will be employed. No sexism. Just word economy.

She got her looks from her father. He was a plastic surgeon.
– Groucho Marx

1
SNAPSHOT of the
BIG PICTURE

Considering Cosmetic Surgery?

- Wondering what to expect?

- What you would look like?

- Think you want it but a bit frightened by the prospect?

- Not sure if it is for you because you have not yet researched it?

- Need some help?

- Some concise, to-the-point information?

- Would you like to have an expert, an advisor at your side to coach you and demystify the process of deciding, "*go*" or "*no go*"?

If yes is your answer to all or most of these seven questions, you hold the the guiding light in your hands. **Let this book be your coach, your personal consultant.** It can ease the way for you. It will make the decision-making process much easier.

You do not even have to buy this book to get an overview of the book's content. It is right here, up front, in this first chapter. An easy way to help you decide whether or not to buy the book. No charge; Chapter 1 is on me.

It will take only ten minutes. If you are at your favorite bookstore, pull up a comfortable chair, grab a cup of coffee, sit and relax a bit. Thumb through this chapter. I am going to give you a sneak preview, a glimpse of what the rest of the chapters will expand upon.

I shall let *you* decide if the book is important for you, if its advice is meaningful, and if you think there is value here. *I'll even share my 16 biggest secrets with you, right now:*

THE 16 MOST IMPORTANT COSMETIC SURGERY SECRETS

Secret #1. Many statisfied cosmetic surgery patients "don't talk." Some of your relations and friends have had something done, but they won't necessarily tell you.

Secret #2. Doctors are flooding into cosmetic surgery. Many lack proper training. Some are incompetent.

Secret #3. Selecting a cosmetic surgeon can be a walk through a minefield. DO YOUR HOMEWORK.

Secret #4. The doctor you want is called a super-specialist—he practices cosmetic surgery *exclusively*.

Secret #5. Many consultations focus on selling, not teaching. When is a "free" consultation too expensive?

Secret #6. A surgeon's "before" and "after" album is filled with clues. You should see lots of photos—and they must be "photographically honest."

Secret #7. Know the 15 smartest questions to ask any cosmetic surgeon.

Secret #8. A consultation without computer imaging has limited value. You need to see, on a computer screen, what you will look like "after."

Secret #9. Fees are negotiable. Know the ropes.

Secret #10. The facility in which you have your procedure done can be as important as who is doing it!

Secret #11. Combining a trip to an exotic location with cosmetic surgery may be a less-than-perfect mix.

> The good physician knows his patients through and through, and his knowledge is bought dearly. Time, sympathy and understanding must be lavishly dispensed, but the reward is to be found in that personal bond which forms the greatest satisfaction of the practice of medicine. One of the essential qualities of the clinician is interest in humanity, for the secret of the care of the patient is in caring for the patient.
>
> **–Francis Weld Peabody, MD, Lecture to Harvard Medical Students, 1927**

Secret #12. Know the difference between an anesthesiologist and an anesthetist. Only one is a medical doctor.

Secret #13. High fees don't necessarily mean better results. Low fees are not always a bargain.

Secret #14. Your chances of post-surgical complications can be reduced by understanding your doctor's philosophy on "aftercare."

Secret #15. Aspirin, herbs, even vitamins can influence your risk during surgery. Be sure to know what to avoid.

Secret #16. There is a responsible answer or solution for every concern, worry and reservation.

Yes, I am "giving it away, free." But that is not an issue for me. What is important is that you get a sense of how very unique and important my insider information is. I am offering to share this with you if you have any interest in improving your appearance.

INSIDER'S INSIGHT

Asking For A Referral?
Here's A Shortcut To The Top Doctors

When asking a friend, doctor or other source for a referral for cosmetic surgery, be specific. Don't say: "Can you give me the name of a great plastic surgeon?" or "Know a good, reputable cosmetic surgeon?"

That's not specific enough. In today's world of doctors, find a superspecialist— one who is an expert in the procedure you want.

If you are considering changing your nose, the wise "Insider's" question is: "Who's known for great noses?" For body liposuction: "Who has the most experience in liposuction?"

Go straight to a superspecialist.

-RK

It may be that when you finish reading this chapter, you will have learned enough to conclude that cosmetic surgery is not for you. And that is fine; as good as cosmetic surgery is for those who have it, it is not for everyone. That will be your choice.

In our practice, it is not the right thing for about 20 percent of the patients who consult with me. One of five. I do not want to deflate a patient's dream and often they will describe my respectful decline as "a disappointment." Rather, I am acting professionally by giving them a responsible, realistic, and honest opinion. Doctor and patient must be on the same page and I will help you level the playing field so you can make a decision with confidence. If you are considering cosmetic surgery, selecting your doctor will be one of the most important decisions of your life. And if it is inappropriate for a man or woman to have a procedure, I shall be best serving those who sit in front of me by giving them my best opinion, an answer based on my years of experience, not an answer they would prefer to hear.

> **Most people don't come to a plastic surgeon wanting to look like someone else. Most people still want to look like themselves, but better.**
>
> **-Garry Brody, MD, USC Professor of Clinical Surgery in *USC Health*, Spring 2001**

I now tell you what I tell such patients: I enjoy doing surgery. It is my life's work and obviously, it is the only way I earn my living. But *my first obligation to you is to give my best; not self-serving, opinion. And sometimes, that boils down to one word: "Don't." Don't if your health is not satisfactory. Don't if even a slight risk of a poor outcome or complication is unacceptable. And don't if you are not certain you really want cosmetic surgery.*

That is how I have done it during 25 years of consulting with over ten thousand prospective patients. Skeptics may scoff at hearing of my telling patients—despite their pleadings—that I do not accept the fee and operate if my heart is not in it. But that is how this doctor practices. It is about integrity—not money—because one, or two, or ten more cases a year will not make a difference in my lifestyle. But, doing surgery without the comfort of knowing that I am doing the right thing would push me over an ethical line I choose not to cross. I prefer to sleep well.

The Perils of Cosmetic Surgery

A middle-aged woman is in a terrible accident and is rushed to the hospital. On the way there, her vital signs fail. The doctors are able to revive her, but while she is gone, she sees God and he tells her she has 40 more years to live.

Since she is in the hospital, and knowing she is going to be around for a while, she decides to use the stay for self-improvement. She has a facelift, an eyelid lift, and a nose job. She gets released from the hospital and, as she crosses the street, she is run over by a truck and killed.

When she sees God again, she says to him, "I thought you said I had 40 years to live"!

To which God replies, "I'm sorry...I didn't recognize you."

If you conclude that you want cosmetic surgery, I strongly encourage you to go into this with eyes wide open. *You want to do it right the first time.*

When performed correctly, cosmetic surgery can transform your life. However, if you are a deluded optimist, too-trusting, do not use good judgment, or even if your expectations are unreasonable or incorrect, you will be disappointed.

I am going to tell it as it is; the good and the bad and the not-too-pleasant. I'll share some possibilities and potentials, but will also reveal some pitfalls that you never thought about. They are all important. And that is why you will be challenged to do two things: look at yourself in the mirror, and look at the entire subject of cosmetic surgery, because many factors must be considered to give you the insight and result you want.

This Book Will Answer Your #1 Question:
What Can I Really Expect?

Secrets of a Beverly Hills Cosmetic Surgeon **is written for those of you who want straight talk.** If you will come with me on the journey we are about to begin, I guarantee I will help you decide if cosmetic surgery is right—or not right—for *you*.

Should you decide that either the time is not right or, for whatever personal reason, you are not committed to undergoing surgery, you can learn about popular nonsurgical alternatives. They are not as powerful, but they work: skin care products and in-office medical treatments that are minimally invasive. You will have a taste of how today's cosmetic surgeons and their allies can help you improve your appearance and slow the clock.

This is a mini-encyclopedia of self-improvement. A menu of treatments from light to heavy, from simple office procedures to more elaborate surgical operations. This is the first behind-the-scenes peek at American cosmetic surgery from one of its own, a bona fide insider, not a professional writer on assignment. An authoritative exposé of this much-discussed—but poorly understoodspecialty a primer on how you can safely navigate through what is the best way for you to obtain the best possible result. By the last page of the book, you will know what you want—and what you do not want—and hopefully, will thank me for the advice.

PATIENT COMMENTARY

This procedure was something I had contemplated for quite a number of years, but I always found a good reason/excuse for not going ahead with it. It was a simple, painless procedure that I had built up in my mind until it became an intimidating prospect involving a huge expense and lots of pain and discomfort. I couldn't have been more wrong. I didn't even take so much as an aspirin while I was recuperating and I was really surprised at how little bruising and swelling was involved. My first thought when I saw my nose after the surgery was "I can't believe I waited all those years!" I still think that when I look in the mirror. I am lucky to have found you when I did, as I can't imagine still walking around with my old nose.

So thank you again, Dr. Kotler! You (and my new nose) have made such a positive impact in my life.

-Heidi, student

The Good, the Bad and the Ugly

For more than a quarter of a century I have been privileged to participate in one of man's more fascinating surgical advances—a gift to himself—the improvement of his appearance. It is an honor to have been chosen by over eight thousand patients to be the doctor who would make a profound and positive change in their lives. In a world where many discretionary purchases and indulgences have a limited lifespan and importance, cosmetic surgery outlasts most, carrying lifelong internal satisfaction.

In less than one generation cosmetic surgery has become an accepted, mainstream undertaking for millions. According to the American Society of Plastic Surgeons, "Surgical and nonsurgical cosmetic surgery procedures in the United States increased 31 percent from 1992 to 2000." Americans are expected to have 8 million cosmetic procedures this year. Its expanding popularity reflects these advances:

> **Any good plastic surgeon is and must be a psychologist, whether he would have it so or not. When you change a man's face you almost invariably change his future. Change his physical image and nearly always you change the man—his personality, his behavior—and sometimes even his basic talents and abilities.**
>
> **-Maxwell Maltz, MD, FICS, author *Psycho-Cybernetics***

- **Expansion of capability**—new solutions for previously unimprovable conditions.

- **Better results** – natural appearing, not "fake" or artificial.

- **Greater longevity of procedures**—today, there is no reason for a facelift to last only two or three years.

- **Reduction in surgical and anesthesia risks**—through the development of both new equipment and refinement of techniques, risks to patients continue to decrease.

- **Shortened operating times**—this translates to a safer procedure and significantly lower fees, opening the door of opportunity to prospective patients who thought they could not afford cosmetic surgery.

- **Minimized recovery time**—patients can return to work in seven to fourteen days; a decided savings in time and money.

Yet, despite these impressive improvements, poor quality cosmetic surgery still exists. While it is a challenge even for me to spot well-done (natural-appearing) cosmetic surgery, it is easy to spot the "unnatural" work. Whether I am walking down Rodeo Drive in Beverly Hills, Michigan Avenue in Chicago, or Fifth Avenue in New York or even Illinois Avenue in Green Lake, Wisconsin, I have noticed the overdone, too-scooped, too-short, nostrils-flaring nose job; or the overtightened, overpulled, walking-through-a-wind-tunnel facelift. Instinctively, I wince. I'm sorry an opportunity for success was missed. In the right hands, our specialty can do better—and does so every day.

A MOTHER'S COMMENTARY

I feel so badly concerning the results of my daughter's nose surgery. It was done by the Chairman of the Department at one of the local medical schools. Only afterward did I find out that most of his time was spent doing reconstructive surgery, not cosmetic surgery, and that particularly he had very little experience doing nasal surgery. My assumption that the Department Chairman at a university was the best person to do the procedure was very poor.

–Mother of teenage patient at consultation for correction of a poorly performed nasal surgery

People are often frightened away from cosmetic surgery as a result of these botched jobs. Unfortunately, some prospective patients have deferred consulting about a cosmetic procedure because of rumors, or first-hand accounts shared by friends or family members of (avoidable) pain and suffering.

These negatives raise a question: *is there a common factor responsible for (a) poor results that some people sustain, (b) the inappropriate, unfounded fears and skepticism that prevent others from achieving their wish for an improvement in appearance? What is wrong? What is the problem?*

The answer, the diagnosis, is lack of adequate, correct information. More and better information is needed: ideally insider information—from an expert, from a source working daily in the trenches of the specialty. Sound advice, parallel to what I seek when choosing professionals for my family or myself. I do not know very much about the inner workings of the architectural, accounting or legal professions. But 35 years after receiving my medical degree, I do know about my profession. Some cosmetic surgery books chronicle individual patient experiences, and others delve deeply into the technical aspects and minutiae of every major and minor procedure. No book, however, has ever revealed the inner workings of this specialty. The culture, the politics, the interspecialty rivalries. And the biggest problem: *the wrong surgeons doing cosmetic surgery.*

> **According to the licensing laws of most states, any licensed physician, regardless of training and experience, may declare himself a plastic surgeon. For that matter, any licensed physician may limit his practice and declare himself a practitioner of any specialty he may select.**
>
> **-Kurt J. Wagner, MD and Gerald Imber, MD, authors,** *Beauty by Design*

This is the first behind-the-scenes peek at American cosmetic surgery from one of its own, a bona fide insider, not a professional writer on assignment. An authoritative exposé of this much-discussed—but poorly understood—specialty. A primer on how you can safely navigate through what is the best way for you to obtain the best possible results.

In cosmetic surgery, there should be only excellence. After all, this specialty is about results, and the results are seen by all. I believe the percentage of unhappy experiences is too high, despite the availability of enough sophisticated practitioners. The glitz, glamour, and inane celebrity-slanted TV and magazine stories, have displaced the meaningful, dispassionate advice needed to make a wise consumer decision. While cosmetic surgery is not a frequent undertaking, it cries out for the same thoughtful, objective analysis as any major purchase. You want to do it well; a poor result cannot necessarily be corrected.

PATIENT COMMENTARY

I consulted with the doctor who said he 'did not really like doing nasal surgery, but would do it for me.' Why would I ever want him to 'do it for me' if he was not happy doing it?

-Carole, businesswoman, California

Since cosmetic surgery is always elective, you have the luxury of time. Time to do the research, the study, the investigation, so you do it right the first time. What I am telling you is that such a search is not quick, nor simple. You are going to have to dig a bit. You are going to have to work. Once again, that old maxim that your parents told you applies: "You get out of something what you put into it." While it is quick and effortless to open your *Yellow Pages* and call the first doctor with the most eye-grabbing ad, I submit that you will not be doing yourself a favor, but rather a bit of dice-rolling. Are long shot odds acceptable to you? If so, I suggest the racetrack. Otherwise, read on.

> **The general stigma surrounding cosmetic plastic surgery as something done only by the vain and rich is vanishing.**
>
> **-Walter Erhardt, MD American Society of Plastic Surgeons**

Mine is a rather unique specialty and an uncommon business. Consider this: Cosmetic surgery is a distinct medical specialty, provided by physicians but, unlike all other specialties, cosmetic surgery does not treat illness. Cosmetic surgeons often have more professional interaction with hair stylists and makeup artists than they do with other physicians.

Cosmetic surgery is a learned profession, but operates more like a business, prospering through marketing, advertising, and price competition. But the fees are inconsistent. For the buyer trying to correlate price with the usual variables of quality and service, the search is perplexing, indeed. Further complicating doctor selection is that today's cosmetic surgeons —from varying educational and training backgrounds, and different specialties—purport to deliver the same services. This is "specialty overlap," and it is explained in **Chapter 3, Selecting the Right Surgeon**. This competition between specialties for the same work makes it harder to select a cosmetic surgeon than it is to choose an electrician. And, this confusion is worsening for you, the consumer. More and more doctors—disheartened and demoralized by the depersonalization of managed care served up by

> **81 percent of 680 workers surveyed by the American Academy of Facial Plastic and Reconstructive Surgery say they would tell co-workers they have had a nose job; only 71 percent would tell friends.**
>
> **Wall Street Journal, December 5 2001**

uncaring, profit-driven insurance companies—are now moving into cosmetic surgery. This doctor flight is a big concern to those of us in medical education.

Cosmetic surgery, wrapped in hope and packaged with excitement, is too often unwisely driven by emotion. The prospective patient can be confused by media coverage that can be poorly researched and sensation-oriented. The checkout line at your grocery store is littered with the latest, enticing celebrity exposés.   But there is no meaningful information for those eager to gather solid facts about the specialty.

Ironically, the people who can best help you understand this road less traveled are those who have had cosmetic surgery. However, many patients do not disclose their surgery. Your co-worker returning from vacation looking "rested" may give credit to a "sleepy little spot" she found rather than the surgeon she visited. How can you get an education when the voices of experience are silent?

> **At one point, I was called the Queen of Plastic Surgery. I did bring it out of the closet. After I talked about all my tucks and jobs, people opened up about theirs. I would be sitting on the couch on the Tonight Show, and someone would lean over and say, "I just had my eyes done" or whatever. I became the clearinghouse for everyone, because I knew all the answers. The surgeons loved me. I loved demystifying.**
>
> **-Phyllis Diller quoted in *Time*, June 2001**

The bottom line is that the consumer has nowhere to go. The media talks too much drivel, the veterans may not talk at all and specialty overlap is confusing. This realization inspired me to share the information I have gathered over 35 years as a physician about what some people still consider a "closet" subject. Who better to tell it to you like it is?

This insight is why this book is my personal mission. I see no reason to keep any of this information secret— cosmetic surgery is too good and too important, but only when done properly. *I want to help you avoid the unfortunate result—whether it be overdone, underdone, or burdened with complications.* Although you need not learn the surgical technicalities of taking a bump off the nose or sculpting the neck or removing a wrinkle, you can

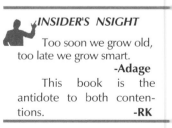

INSIDER'S NSIGHT

Too soon we grow old, too late we grow smart.
        -Adage
This book is the antidote to both contentions.   **-RK**

learn the formula for finding the most qualified professionals who will do the best possible job for you.

With this book my objective are:

- **To present important informatio**n—known within our specialty—and unknown to the public.

- **To outline a clear, rational methodology** by which you can research cosmetic surgery and choose the best doctor to serve you.

- **To provide you an easy-to-follow manual** and specific tools (smart questions) with which to conduct your search.

My experience as a surgeon began as a resident trainee in 1968. The length and depth of my personal history as a physician qualifies me to help you better understand the inner workings of today's cosmetic surgery because the world of medicine is different from what existed when I opened my practice. You need to learn—within the context of the rapid changes that have visited the medical profession—how this new health care climate has created a fresh set of challenges for physicians. **Managed Care has driven many doctors to retool and begin doing cosmetic surgery.** But that migration often translates to inconsistent patient results given the absence of formalized and adequate training—under expert super-vision—heretofore the hallmark of medical education. Yes, it may say "Plastic Surgery" or "Cosmetic Surgery" on the office door, but you must find out more about the kind of plastic or cosmetic surgery the doctor performs, and his qualifications to do it.

> I don't know how things are in California today, but in Florida, they are awful. We have family practitioners and ophthalmologists doing full body liposuction, anesthesiologists doing breast augmentation and oral surgeons, dermatologists and ophthalmologists doing face lifts—all quite legally! It seems everyone wants to be a plastic surgeon. I can understand since it is a wonderful and very gratifying profession...and the "cash on the barrelhead" nature of cosmetic surgery is certainly attractive in this day of declining reimbursement from third-party insurers. What I cannot understand is the pell-mell rush to discard our long-established residency training system in order to allow a few individuals to circumvent the formal training process and call themselves plastic surgeons.
>
> -Richard T. Bosshardt, MD, FACS
> *Bulletin of the American College of Surgeons*, May 2001

Choosing an amateur or rookie without the right resume is a recipe for failure. Your road to a safe, comfortable experience and "great result" will take you on a specialist recognition course. You will learn how to pick the most appropriate and highly skilled doctor. Of all your decisions, this is the most critical. Stumble here and you are down the wrong road. You will learn about superspecialists—the specialist's specialist, if you will. Doctors at the pinnacle of training, experience, focus and performance. The superstars of the medical profession.

To find these superstars, you will have to do some sifting and winnowing. But I shall make it smoother and easier for you. In **Chapter 3, Selecting the Right Surgeon,** you will learn how to eliminate second-string players by one short call to an office or a quick peek at a professional biography. That way, you won't waste precious time and your hard-earned dollars in a consultation with the wrong doctor.

INSIDER'S INSIGHT

Superspecialist For Your Auto But not For Yourself?

Consider the importance of focus and specialization, think about that certified car mechanic who works only on your imported car, for example. Given a choice between the corner gas station repairman who claims to "fix everything," and the factory trained technician, who will be likely to fix your car the first time? Today's automobiles have an average of 15,000 moving parts. Is it possible for any mechanic to become an expert in the inner workings of dozens of car models? Doesn't *your* human body—the only one you'll ever own—deserve the most specialized repairman?

-RK

You sort and select by knowing the smart questions to ask at each level of research, up to and through the consultation. Treat the consultation as an interview. While the surgeon is evaluating you medically, you are evaluating him for an appropriate match. Study this book well, my friend, and you will earn an A+ in Cosmetic Surgery Consultation. And, you should fight for that A+ because this is so important to you. You want no regrets, no remorse, no whining that you did not do enough homework. You want the best possible result. Because when your cosmetic surgery result is good, a big, wide smile looks back at you from your mirror.

Look Closely at That *Before and After* Album

Once you are savvy enough to consult with superspecialists (the ones who perform cosmetic surgery exclusively), how do you then choose among this already select talent pool? You begin by critically examining before and after photos. You must look at them as analytically as an auction house examines a work of art. I will coach you and teach you visual analysis. You will know how to use the practice's "before and after" albums as a measurement of what you are buying: the doctor's talent as displayed in his art form.

Why Not See What You'll Look Like?

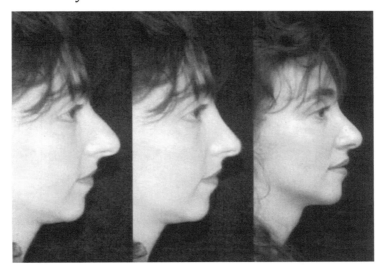

Computer imaging, three views. (1) Left: "before." (2) Middle: "computer imaged preview." (3) Right: "final result: nasal surgery and chin augmentation."*

If you've been tempted to try cosmetic surgery but have always held back, what I've described may have piqued your interest sufficiently so that you're ready to cross the threshold. In that case, you'll want to devote a good deal of time and energy to choosing the right surgeon. I've had some experience with all this, and I know how important it is to make that choice, yet how difficult it can sometimes be to choose wisely.

-Kathy Keeton, author
Longevity: the Science of Staying Young

Top quality, informative, valuable consultations must include a computer-generated transformation of your "before" photo into a satisfactory "after." Otherwise, it is all guesswork. Who buys something without seeing it? You don't want to sign up for a nose job, facelift, or breast augmentation without knowing what you will look like after the surgery. Today's remarkable computer technology can show you a preview, a realistic prediction of the new you. It answers that lurking question: "What will I look like…after?" And a conscientious cosmetic surgeon tries to obtain even better results.

Some Operating Rooms Are Safer than Others

Would you like to know if the facility meets demanding safety standards? If it has a medical *"Good Housekeeping*® **Seal of Approval"**? Every day you enter buildings that require an occupancy-safety license to

---

* The above patient after seeing the computer image of the predicted result, opted, just before surgery, to improve her profile by adding the chin augmentation.

keep the doors open. You then ride up and down in elevators that are regularly inspected and licensed. You cannot operate a potentially dangerous 4,000-pound machine—called an automobile—without an operator's license.

Doesn't it make sense that a facility where you are deliberately rendered unconscious—and therefore helpless—be credentialed and meet strict code standards for structural integrity, fire protection and even earthquake resistance? Big risks will be avoided by knowing the difference between an unlicensed, unaccredited, never-inspected facility, large or small, and a state-licensed, U.S. government-certified, independently accredited, specialized outpatient surgery center, or a fully accredited hospital. There are accepted guidelines for evaluating surgical facilities. You must know about them.

Don't Forget to Ask About Anesthesia

While most people focus on the cosmetic surgery itself, they fail to realize that the big risk is not the "cutting and sewing"—it is the anesthetic. That is why I shall teach you the difference between professionals who aid the surgeon by administering the anesthetic. *Do you know the difference between an anesthetist and an anesthesiologist?* The former are nurses, the latter are physician-specialists. Think about who will be at the controls during your surgery.

Insider Information Is Precious
When You Discuss Dollars

I shall level the playing field and arm you with negotiation strategies that will save you money. Here is a sample: understanding that it makes good business sense for a doctor to operate on two or more patients (not at the same time, of course), at a reduced "group rate" can translate into significant savings for you and a surgery partner. The efficiency of this practice converts to a discounted fee; more on this in **Chapter 6, "About Fees" and Chapter 10, "Erasing Mental Blocks."**

Having your procedure on a "stand by" basis or opting for prepayment can also help lower your cost. Since the individual cash outlay can be $5,000 to $10,000, a saving of 15 to 20 percent equals hundreds or thousands of dollars. Good business for your doctor can be great savings for you. Do you wonder how cosmetic surgeons price their services? And, one of the secrets that may surprise you, is that the *most skilled superspecialists are not necessarily the most expensive.* **Chapter 6** reveals the explanation.

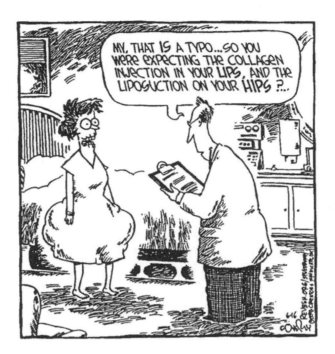

You Don't Want the Ball to Be Dropped
Before or After Surgery

The practice you want will give you old-fashioned, one-on-one, attentive care. Top practices prepare you for everything and anticipate your needs.

The best cosmetic surgery practices provide for your total care from beginning to end:

- *Make sure you are fit for surgery —* healthy.

- *Give you written instructions* telling you what to expect, before and after, and answer all questions.

- *Provide routine medications and supplies.* Your needs are anticipated.

- *Make house calls, if necessary.* (Yes, you read that correctly).

While cosmetic surgeons do not cure cancer, give you a new liver, or replace a worn-out hip, we are still medical doctors, not—as some would paint us—highly-educated beauticians. Many of us still know how to give that now-elusive patient care. The best practices give it. These are the practices you should seek. I can show you the way.

If you have relatives or friends in the cosmetic surgery world, you are fortunate because you automatically have insider information. They will lead you down the right path. But if you do not have a brother, cousin or best friend who is a cosmetic surgeon, you are still in luck; I shall fill the pathfinder role for you. The knowledge you are about to gain is important; cosmetic surgery—despite the hype—is not trivial. It is not casual surgery. It is about your body. There is a bit more complexity to cosmetic surgery than you thought. You must be vigilant. Forewarned is forearmed.

The most important secret from this Beverly Hills cosmetic surgeon is that there are too many secrets about cosmetic surgery. Too much hype, too many silly, shallow celebrity stories, and too little practical, important, even life-saving information.

Appearance is a subjective and emotionally charged subject. However, changing your appearance surgically should never be based solely on emotion. Instead, there is a prescribed methodology to selecting a proper surgeon, opting for the appropriate procedure, and choosing a comfortable, safe location.

My hope is that this book will influence your approach by erasing myths, misconceptions, and misrepresentations, making your research process unintimidating, efficient, and satisfying. I want you to enjoy the best possible result reflected in your mirror.

Dental panel targets cometic surgery

HEALTH: The illegal practice by oral surgeons has been ignored but now faces probable penalties.

By KIMBERLY KINDY
The Orange County Register

Oral surgeons performing illegal facial cosmetic surgery in California will likely be punished with large fines, jail time, permanent marks on their records — even the loss of their dental licenses.

The state Dental Board of Examiners is expected Friday to approve a list of proposed crackdowns.

"We are sending a very strong message," said Dr. Peter Hartman, a general dentist and dental board member. "I don't think anyone who is performing these procedures should be confused about where we stand on the issue and what might happen."

Oral and maxillofacial surgeons typically hold dental but not medical licenses. Some also have medical degrees, meaning they can perform the procedures.

The procedures in question are those that venture too far from the jaw and mouth and aren't related to dentistry.

For years, the dental board has looked the other way as some oral surgeons performed eyelid surgery, neck liposuction, even face lifts. It has investigated only when something went wrong and someone complained.

The board went after the oral surgeons — who frequently advertise their illegal work — after a series of stories in The Orange County Register revealed that the practice is widespread.

"Until now, there was no real incentive for them to change their behavior," said state Sen. Liz Figueroa, D-Fremont, who chairs a committee that oversees the dental board. "This puts them on notice. People are watching now, and there are consequences."

▶ **BOARD:** Oral surgeons to be put on notice. **News 14**

Orange County, CA newspaper reveals crackdown on dental specialists performing facial cosmetic surgery. January 8, 2000.
(Notice their typo in headline.)

The next chapter—which may be a bit of a shocker—is titled, **"The Terrible Truth About Some Cosmetic Surgeons."** But, better to know sooner than later, before rather than after.

Why Do Some Celebrities Look So Bad After Cosmetic Surgery?

That's a question often asked by prospective patients. The common assumption is that money, power and access should automatically guarantee garnering top cosmetic surgery talent. Not always.

I see three reasons why some celebrities look so bad after cosmetic surgery. Bad luck is not one of them.

1. **Bad decision making.** Celebrities—like the rest of us—are not immune from making bad purchasing decisions. They are not anointed with special wisdom because of their fame. They may not do enough research to sort out the most talented practitioners for their particular needs. Or they rely on a manager or advisor to conduct the search. Off the screen, away from the studio, they own no magic, no divining rod to lead them to the right offices. They need to do their homework; just like you.

2. **Not knowing when to stop.** When you see obvious and overdone cosmetic surgery on the face of a celebrity, it usually announces that they did not know when to stop. They kept going beyond reason. Perhaps the celebs were unwisely shooting for perfection, for immortality. But they are on a hopeless chase. Regardless of who is famous or otherwise, the same rules of life govern us all.

3. **A cosmetic surgeon who falls into the celebrity trap**. He, too, drops common sense. He forgets that mantra his mentors hammered into his memory bank: *"The pursuit of perfection is the ultimate enemy of good."* Overdoing is always worse than underdoing. That it is easier to add on later, but almost impossible to "put back that which you took off." But why does an ordinarily objective and wise doctor temporarily discard the sound advice his teachers gave him? Because, he, too, has a chance to be a celebrity, however vicarious. An opportunity to bask in that special glow we Americans are so good at fostering is often too hard to pass up.

Media personalities are attractive, smart and charming; that is how they reached their level of success and fame. They can be very manipulative, very convincing in their arguments. Isn't that their craft? That is why, it is hard to say "no" to the lady or gentleman sitting in front of you whose face may be recognized by billions of people. And, perhaps subconsciously, the doctor wants to say yes, wants to satisfy this important person, to ingratiate himself, to join the club, to be part of that special world. It can be heady stuff.

Consulting with famous people is very difficult. I have been there many times. The doctor must harness his best instincts, his purest motives, his strongest common sense to do the right thing for every patient regardless of status. Not for himself, his ego, his office's "wall of fame" photo display, or his bank account.

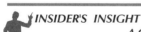 *INSIDER'S INSIGHT*

A Celebrity's Cosmetic Surgery Disaster

Years ago comedian Totie Fields died because of a cosmetic misadventure. Knowing that Totie was obese and diabetic should have been a bright enough red flag for any conscientious cosmetic surgeon to decline to operate.

Totie developed a blocked artery which led to to her complications, snowballing to her tragic premature death.

I share this to remind you that the first decision about cosmetic surgery is whether or not it is right to do it. In the "reasons not to do it" column, at the top, always stands: "Medical condition(s); too risky."

I urge you to consult with a doctor whose practice is not a cosmetic surgery conveyer belt. You want a doctor who thinks first and operates second.

-RK

It is the duty, and ought to be the pleasure, of age and experience to warn and instruct youth . . .What man of common humanity, having, by good luck, missed being engulfed in a quagmire or quicksand, will withhold from his neighbors a knowledge of the peril…?
-William Cobbett, "Advice to Young Men and
(incidentally) To Young Women
in the Middle and Higher Ranks of Life," 1829

2
The TERRIBLE TRUTH About Some COSMETIC SURGEONS

Secret: Doctors are flooding into cosmetic surgery. Many lack proper training.

Even more patients end up with less than satisfactory results because of the ineptitude of the surgeons they chose to perform some cosmetic surgery operations. Cosmetic surgery remains a largely unregulated business and many physicians who are performing plastic or cosmetic surgery receive their formal training in another specialty.

Dermatologists perform eyelid surgery; gynecologists do liposuction; ear, nose and throat specialists do breast implants. Merely by taking a weekend course, physicians can hang out a new shingle as a cosmetic surgeon. Often, they operate out of poorly equipped offices with insufficiently trained staff. Such physicians often attract patients by offering cut-rate deals and bargain basement prices.

The industry is rife with misleading advertising including those claiming board certification or suggesting an industry seal of approval. These doctors place what appear to be informational articles about themselves and their services in flick magazines but which are actually paid advertisements meant to appeal to high-income clients.

-Joyce Nash, Ph.D. author
*What Your Doctor Can't
Tell You About Cosmetic Surgery*

JUST BECAUSE A DOCTOR PERFORMS COSMETIC SURGERY DOES NOT MEAN HE IS COMPETENT. A doctor should not just "start doing cosmetic surgery" anymore than a commercial pilot starts flying a space shuttle. He needs training. He needs supervised experience under an expert.

Unqualified cosmetic surgeons can establish a practice in two different ways:

- Entrance from another specialty without adequate "re-training" or

- Completion of an accredited residency training program that lacks specific training in cosmetic surgery

> **Many physicians are now turning to cosmetic surgery as a way to supplement their income. Is this good for the quality of care we deliver to a cosmetic surgery patient? I think not.**
>
> **-Rod J. Rohrich, MD**
> **The journal *Plastic and Reconstructive Surgery*, June 2001**

The breakdown of traditional specialty boundaries makes it more challenging to select the appropriate cosmetic surgeon for your needs. Some doctors are lax about gaining enough training, while others become highly skilled. Some examples of successful transitions are:

- Body liposuction was not devised by a cosmetic surgeon, but rather by a French gynecologist—and it was later refined by an American doctor, board certified in both internal medicine and dermatology.

- One of the most prominent hair transplant specialists in the country originally practiced psychiatry.

- The father of modern cosmetic nasal surgery was a Berlin orthopedic surgeon.

The migration of some specialists into cosmetic surgery is parallel to the deregulation of the airline industry and public utilities—you might have more choices, but it is difficult to choose wisely.

> **Facing a decline in earnings, many physicians have eagerly added body contouring with liposuction to their office practices. Many are well trained, but some physicians have launched into office liposuction with minimal or inadequate education and training. A physician who lacks hospital surgical privileges, or one who already treats obese patients for related conditions, may be tempted to add high demand, cash-producing liposuction to his or her repertoire.**
>
> **-Fredrick M. Grazer, MD**
> **Plastic and Reconstructive Surgery**

Media Observations on Doctors Transferring to Cosmetic Surgery

Leslie Vreeland, an experienced investigative reporter, wrote in *American Health* in 1992, ". . . you must make sure your surgeon is qualified. Thanks to an explosion in the number of doctors entering the field, the odds that you will choose the wrong one may be greater today than ever before." Vreeland quotes Mark Gorney, MD, a plastic surgeon practicing at that time in San Francisco, and senior examiner for the American Board of Plastic Surgery: "Cosmetic surgery is attracting all sorts of people who lack training or scruples. There are now so many of us in this profession, we're almost practicing on each other."

Vreeland noted that while the number of operations done for cosmetic reasons had risen significantly in the prior ten years, "the number of doctors vying for the business had increased even faster." And that article was written a decade ago. Many more have entered the field since then.

How Managed Care Drives Doctors into Cosmetic Surgery

For many physicians, the impediments to providing high quality care for their patients has led to disenchantment, frustration and, frequently, even despair.

Rather than continue the ongoing battle with managed care organizations and other third party payers, many physicians are leaving medicine, retiring early, or changing the focus of their practices, and begin performing only elective procedures, including cosmetic surgery.

-Ronald G. Wheeland, MD
Editorial Perspective,
***Cosmetic Surgery Times,* Jan/Feb 2000**

Revolutionary changes in medical care delivery, as orchestrated by the insurance industry, have altered physician attitudes and career directions. Many—disheartened, disillusioned and disgusted with the duplicity of their insurance company masters—have reluctantly re-evaluated their careers. They have seen one last refuge of independence: cosmetic surgery. The only specialty unburdened by unending paperwork served up by a sinister, maze-like bureaucracy adept at payment delays, payment slashes, or, worse yet, no payment.

So just in case you wanted to know one reason behind that swing to cosmetic surgery—this is the answer from an insider.

Legally, Can Any Licensed Doctor Perform Cosmetic Surgery?   Technically, Yes. Practically, No

> Choosing a good plastic surgeon is not easy. The patient-to-be can expect to hear claims that may be misleading, and the lack of government and peer control is worrisome. Ask physicians about their precise credentials, training, and field of expertise. If advertisements say: "board-certified," find out which board and whether it is accredited by the American Board of Medical specialties. Be aggresive in your questioning. Dr. Norman Cole says: "I am amazed at how few questions people usually ask me about my training and credentials."
>
> -Kathy Keeton, author
> *Longevity, the Science of Staying Young*

Hold on; do not panic. Having heard the media play this tune so often as part of a rating-boosting, sensational story, I must comment. The unstated implication is that a family practitioner, right out of internship, or an allergist, just finishing his specialty training, can start performing liposuction, face-lifts and nose jobs on a whim—*not quite.*

My license to practice is granted by the State of California's Medical Board, the state's regulator. It is a Physician & Surgeon license. So it is for every state's licensed doctors. The license makes no mention of specialty.

> Any licensed M.D. can legally perform cosmetic surgery procedures.
>
> -The American Society of Aesthetic Plastic Surgery

Every doctor's license is general and not specialty-specific because it is impractical for California (84,675 licensed MDs as of January 1, 2002) or any state to oversee professional competence in each of the dozens of specialties, subspecialties, and now, superspecialties. However, using a traditionally wise practice, hospitals and outpatient facilities such as radiology centers, laboratories, and surgery centers where doctors ply their trade have been charged with the background check and credentialing of its practitioners. The system works well because each facility has strict, uniform criteria for granting privileges for specialists to perform their work. The privilege-granting process, after a thorough credentialing and background check, is guided by each specialty's recognized standards.

Example of How the System Works

> Consumers should be able to select a surgeon based on informed choice. Consumers have the right to be fully informed of their doctor's credentials and what they mean. Physicians have an ethical responsibility not to misrepresent their training.
>
> -The American Society for Aesthetic Plastic Surgery

If an orthopedic surgeon applies for privileges at the XYZ Surgery Center, he must present proof of licensure, liability insurance, and a credentials packet that reflects medical schooling, internship, and residency training in the doctor's specialty in this case, orthopedics.

Further, the doctor must submit a list of surgical procedures for which he seeks performance privileges. Assuming his credentials are appropriate (board certification or board eligible in orthopedic surgery, an unrestricted state license, and personal list of procedures falling within standard orthopedic practice), he will be allowed to practice, on a temporary/guest basis, until his skills are deemed satisfactory. Only then will full staff membership be granted allowing him to practice orthopedic surgery at the XYZ Surgery Center.

Here's a "hypothetical" example of how the watchdog system, protects you. Another board certified orthopedic surgeon comes to the same surgery center, with intentions of expanding his orthopedic practice to include liposuction on hips or thighs. He states: "Hey, I can do this. I know the anatomy of the hips and thighs. I have been operating there for years." And indeed, while he is knowledgeable in the anatomy of that area, this alone is not an adequate qualification to begin doing a cosmetic procedure, especially when he admits he has no formal, approved training and no experience.

His application will have to be evaluated, not by the Orthopedic Surgery department but by the Plastic Surgery department. His application will be promptly denied because he does not meet the professional standard of the surgery center: specialty training in the procedure he wishes to perform. Cosmetic surgery on the hip area, such as liposuction, is a procedure that is not listed by his board—the American Board of Orthopedic Surgery—as a procedure within the scope of the specialty. The safeguard to you, the prospective patient, is that an ethical clinic allows only fully-accredited, properly trained professionals to perform specific surgeries.

Besides the moral obligation to protect the public, a hospital or surgery center has a business-driven reason to scrupulously follow the privilege-granting guideline it submitted to inspectors before receiving license, certification or accreditation. Not following these guidelines would disqualify them from government and private insurance payments. This complex system of internal quality control is all "behind the scenes"—for your safety and protection. Ninety-nine percent of the time it works. Ethical surgeons and ethical surgery centers play by the rules: no qualification—no surgery.

Yes, there have been some shocking stories of general practitioners or other untrained, self- proclaimed cosmetic surgeons doing liposuction without proper training and accepted credentials. Because these doctors could not qualify for privileges in a bona fide hospital or surgery center, they have opted to "go underground" and the danger to patients is real.

The rare unscrupulous physician, with no legitimate facility to accept him, retreats to his office or some under-equipped, inadequately staffed, unlicensed, uncredentialed, underground hideout. These inadequate pseudo-clinics are the wrong place for surgery of any kind, and breed problems for the patients that can have a tragic ending.

I can assure you such a scenario is very, very rare. But, as mentioned earlier, my mission is to make sure you are savvy enough not to consider any high-risk shortcuts. These never lead to safety and excellence. By staying "mainstream," you remain safe and you remain distant from danger.

> We created residencies and said, "medicine is so complex that one can really only be educated satisfactorily in a particular area, and to do that one needs to do a residency." But when it comes to aesthetic (cosmetic) surgery, if you take a two-day course in Boca Raton and can get somebody to lie still, you can do an operation. With the reimbursements and benefits of other medical areas deteriorating, we have numerous individuals with all types of training, calling themselves cosmetic surgeons — we have dentists and cardiologists doing it.
>
> What we've done is to cheapen what we spent years creating — the process of residency training. It also cheapens what we do and tells the public that aesthetic (cosmetic) surgery is really just glorified cosmetology —it has no risks and anybody can do it — and that's just not true.
>
> -John Grossman, MD in
> *Cosmetic Surgery Times*, November/December 2000

Although the majority of specialties may not include cosmetic surgery in their practices, enough do so that the lines traditionally drawn between specialties continue to sway and weaken. Prospective patients must be aware of this evolution.

The Training Program Problem

William P. Graham III, MD, former chairman of the American Board of Plastic Surgery, stated in his Carlson Lectureship in 1994 that "Although aesthetic (cosmetic) surgery is absolutely integral to a basic plastic surgery education, it is the fact that the quality of aesthetic training varies greatly among residencies. Training opportunities in aesthetic surgery are not as accessible to the large superspecialized university center as they are to the freestanding facility or small, private hospital. How do we ensure the availability of appropriate aesthetic surgical training to all plastic surgery residents, and what minimum standard should be set for resident experience in aesthetic surgery?"

-from an editorial entitled "Aesthetic Surgical Education: A Personal Perspective" by Stanley A. Klatsky, MD Editor-in-Chief, *Aesthetic Surgery Journal*, November/ December 1999

Until recently, many training programs properly fulfilled their mission. But, today's training programs differ significantly from the programs we enjoyed a generation ago. As a trainee at the University of Illinois in the early 1970s, I had access to a generous stream of patients seeking cosmetic surgery. The university made it very affordable for patients to have surgery performed by surgeons-in-training because the hospital had a plump budget, which included funds for noninsured training cases. Patients paid between $50 and $250 for a single or multiple procedures. This inflow of patients seeking our services allowed many of us to become quite accomplished during our residencies. We graduated both competent and confident in our skills. Our professors felt comfortable sending us out to do cosmetic facial surgery.

> **INSIDER'S INSIGHT**
>
> A more disturbing trend than doctors practicing outside their experience zone is the fundamental breakdown in residency training programs for doctors specifically seeking a cosmetic surgery career.
>
> *-RK*

By contrast, today's residency training programs often work against the aspiring young cosmetic surgeon. First, there is the time constraint of the training period itself. Consider this: The minimum residency requirement for plastic surgeons is only two years. For the entire body. Is this adequate time to master the 137 head-to-toe procedures that the American Board of Plastic and Reconstructive Surgery recognizes as within that specialty's province? In fact, the training focuses on the reconstructive procedures required by accident and tumor victims, not cosmetic surgery patients. Furthermore, since most residency training is held in hospitals, rather than boutique clinics or dedicated cosmetic surgery centers, residents aspiring to be cosmetic surgeons have inadequate training and little access to the cosmetic wing of plastic surgery.

The dilemma is the same for opthalmologists aspiring to perform cosmetic surgery on the eyelid and brow; for head and neck surgeons interested in face and neck cosmetic surgery; and for dermatologists seeking training in cosmetic procedures. Residency focus is on reconstructive—not cosmetic—surgery.

What other barriers exist to proper training and experience before a doctor starts performing cosmetic procedures in practice? One is that *today's more sophisticated and well-informed patients are reluctant to have the procedures performed by novice surgeons-in-training.* They realize that regardless of the amount of supervision, if a doctor-in-training is performing the procedure, his inexperience may negatively influence their result.

Cosmetic Surgery Is *Not* a Hospital-Based Subspecialty

Like other subspecialties of plastic surgery, dermatology, head and neck and ophthalmic surgery, cosmetic surgery lives in an outpatient world. It is not hospital based because the patients do not require hospitalization before or after surgery. This has great significance for trainees who are generally hospital bound. How difficult must it be for a hospital bound cosmetic surgery resident to gain experience in a specialty that is not hospital based? Most highly specialized, full time cosmetic surgeons are found in larger cities, practicing apart from university hospital settings. They practice in either office or outpatient surgery centers. Not in hospitals. Contrary to reconstructive cases, the cosmetic surgeon does not see the patient preoperatively or postoperatively in the hospital. This is a major disadvantage for doctors in training.

Neophytes need to learn the entire menu of the surgical experience. The operating room is only one course. They need exposure on how to interview patients. They must learn "when to operate, and when not to operate." Medical photography and computer imaging are rarely available in an all-purpose university hospital. Learning how to manage patients postoperatively is imperative. Dealing with patient dissatisfaction, post-operative problems and complications mean care is often given for months after surgery. Trainees often change services every two to three months and never get the full benefit of having their work evaluated on a long-term basis. Thus, we must conclude, the university training setting is not a replica of the actual practice world for the cosmetic surgeon.

Ironically, the typical cosmetic surgery patient is not anxious to go to a teaching hospital, but that's where the trainees are based. It offers little privacy, no anonymity, and hospital charges are often prohibitive. Cosmetic surgeons are even less excited about a hospital stay for their patients. The threat of antibiotic-resistant bacteria is a concern with elective surgery, which should be done in a low risk environment. And, overworked hospital nurses are not ideal service providers for the special needs of cosmetic clients; their inherent allegiance is to the sick, not to the vain.

The Uncomfortable Truth About Teaching

By traditional ethics and public insistence (not to mention court rulings), a patient's right to the best care possible must trump the objective of training novices. We want perfection without practice. Yet everyone is harmed if no one is trained for the future. So learning is hidden, behind drapes and anesthesia and the elisions of language. And the dilemma doesn't apply to just residents, physicians in training. The process of learning goes on longer than most people know.

-from "Annals of Medicine
The Learning Curve. Like everyone else, surgeons
need to practice. That's where you come in."
by Atul Gawande, MD
New Yorker, January 28, 2002

The Heavy Hand of Today's Managed Care Economics

The other current major cosmetic surgery training negative is a heavy, cloud-like factor permeating all training programs and it is not healthy for any of us. Hospital budgets—particularily those of teaching hospitals—are severely constricted by managed care's impact.

Community hospitals concentrate on providing services to the quick, uncomplicated, rountine surgical case. They are economically unable to shoulder patients who do not fit within this narrow parameter. The complex cases are shunted to the university's teaching hospitals. Consequently, these are overfollowing with the sickest patients. With full censuses and day and night operating schedules, the harried admissions department has little space for elective cosmetic surgery patients. And already stressed hospital administrators, sweating their thin budgets, do not roll out the Welcome Wagon for long, pro-bono cosmetic training cases that may consume two to three times the operating room time typically allotted to experienced surgeons.

Unfortunately, In Most Residency Programs, Cosmetic Surgery Is Still A Stepchild

Cosmetic surgery rarely finds champions in academia, either. Cosmetic cases are perceived as unimportant, extraneous and irrelevant by the university hierarchy who are dedicated to research and teaching.

Recently, in the classified section of a specialty news magazine, under "Opportunities for Plastic Surgeons" appeared these three ads.

Academic Position
The Section of Plastic Surgery at the University of Kansas Medical Center is seeking an individual to join the full time academic faculty. We are looking for an individual with broad clinical interests. Eligibility for the CAQHS is desirable but not necessary. Applicants must be Board certified or eligible to take the certification exams of the American Board of Plastic Surgery. The individual should be committed to the teaching of Plastic Surgery and clinical and/or basic science research. The University of Kansas is an equal opportunity employer. Interested individuals should contact: W. Thomas Lawrence, MD, Chief, Section of Plastic Surgery, Sutherland Institute, University of Kansas Medical Center, 3901 Rainbow Blvd, Kansas City, Kansas 66160.

Medical school ad seeking faculty.

Seeking BC/BE Plastic Surgeon
BC/BE Plastic Surgeon Associate for busy aesthetic, reconstructive and hand practice in west central Wisconsin. Excellent community with opportunity for growth. Hand fellowship preferred. Reply to Box 2088 c/o *PSN*.

Atlanta Plastic Surgery
Rapidly growing Atlanta private practice seeking an energetic and personable associate who is broadly trained and interested in practicing breast, hand, maxillofacial, microvascular and cosmetic surgery. Competitive salary and benefits offered along with future potential for partnership. Fax resume 404-875-4017.

Private practitioner ads seeking associates.

The university ad does not mention cosmetic surgery. In contrast, the ads placed by private practitioners seeking associates indicate cosmetic (aesthetic) surgery experience as a desirable qualification. This is a disconnect between the aims and interests of training programs and the requirements of the real world of cosmetic surgery.

This is not a good thing! If instructors, and even heads of training programs, are neither qualified nor interested in cosmetic surgery, how skilled will their graduates be? And, how can today's ever-increasing demand be met by these training programs?

I submit to you that university training programs are on one track, and the learning desires of trainees—and the demands of the practice community—are on another track. The tracks are well established and parallel, but, as we learned in geometry, parallel lines never meet.

With the exception of those who pursue cosmetic surgery fellowships after their training residency, the young graduate surgeon is often inadequately prepared to practice cosmetic surgery at the high level of expertise expected by today's patient.

I am aware of several young local surgeons who, although well trained in reconstructive surgery, entered private practice with precious little facial cosmetic surgery experience, particularly in face lifting and nasal surgery. Alas, the aspiring—but neophyte—surgeons had to learn cosmetic surgery "on the job." Uninformed, unwary patients inadvertently became the teaching cases that should have been provided during the formal training period.

It is a matter of buyer beware. As an observant colleague commented: "Some people spend less time researching their face lift than they do selecting a refrigerator or a car." Read on and you will become sufficiently well informed to make a wise and safe decision.

THE ULTIMATE INSIDER'S INSIGHT

I Have Been A Patient, Too!

You know the television ad for that hairpiece company. After you have seen some "before and after" photos of satisfied customers, the president of the company, Sy Sperling, sporting a piece himself, proudly announces: "I'm also a client."

That is a strong testimonial. Sy wears and believes in his company's product.

Well, I am proud to paraphrase Mr. Sperling: I have been a patient, too. Not of myself, of course, but I have had cosmetic surgery. And I tell you, frankly, that it is one of the best things I have ever done. Yes, it took some time from work and there was some dollar outlay. My wife was skeptical—before—but not after. My friends "weren't certain you needed it."

But I knew what I wanted and I never regretted the decision. But what this means to you is that I know what it is like to be a patient. I know what it is like to sit in the patient's chair across from the doctor I am consulting with. I, too, know what it is like to be concerned about anesthesia. I have been through the recovery phase, including stitch removal. I have had the whole course as a patient.

The experience as a cosmetic surgery patient has made me a better physician and helped me refine the service aspects of my practice. I may be more sensitive to the issue of attentive postoperative care and pain medication. I, too, had to face issues of how quickly I could resume my sports activities and return to work (six days after nasal cosmetic surgery).

It was a positive experience. But maybe it was a little easier for me because, as you now understand, I had insider information.

-RK

The story may be apocryphal, but it's said that in order to choose a nose surgeon, one high-placed Hollywood wife, who wanted a very conservative operation, gave a luncheon for a dozen friends—each of whom had had a nose job—and compared the results.

-Joan Kron, author
Lift: Wanting, Fearing and Having a Face-Lift

3
SELECTING the RIGHT SURGEON

Secret: Selecting a cosmetic surgeon can be a walk through a minefield.

Tips on Doing Your Homework

COSMETIC SURGERY IS ELECTIVE (not essential to life) surgery. You have the luxury of time to make the best decision possible. The challenge you will face is finding, managing and interpreting all the information available. Should you listen to friends who have had cosmetic surgery? Do you count the certificates on the doctor's wall? Is a Harvard diploma more significant than a UCLA diploma? Is a fancy office important? Could medical colleagues provide clues? Are socialite cosmetic surgeons the best? Is a fresh-in-practice doctor a good choice because he's "up on the latest"? Is it a favorable sign if the doctor drives a Rolls Royce? The answers may surprise you.

Developing the ability to select competent physicians is an integral part of becoming an educated and intelligent consumer of medical care. When you are placing your physical and mental well-being in the hands of an individual, it is important to know as much about him as possible. In medicine, as in all other matters in which choices are made, it is important to understand the ground rules and to learn to use them in locating those professionals who can be of greatest assistance to you.

-from *Beauty by Design*,
Kurt J. Wagner, MD, and Gerald Imber, MD

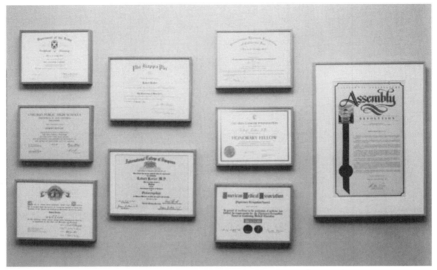

A surgeon's training is long, strenuous and demanding.

You will never ever make a completely objective decision regarding your appearance. This is why one of the most reliable routes for choosing a cosmetic surgeon is through a recommendation from a friend or acquaintance pleased with his or her surgery's result. If a person is willing to share that they have had cosmetic surgery, she will usually be equally willing to discuss the entire experience. Be careful to compare the procedure you are considering with the one they have had. Remember "nose to nose" and "eyelids to eyelids." Don't assume a brilliant eyelift guarantees the expertise demanded for full facelifts.

Excellent sources of referrals are medical personnel—doctors, nurses, hospital staff, technicians, and particularly surgeons, surgical nurses, and anesthesia specialists. Those who actually see the cosmetic surgeon performing his craft in the operating room are the most useful witnesses. You will want to ask about the surgeon's judgment, conduct, and ability. No competent, reputable surgeon ever resents inquiries from any source regarding his professional standing. His most precious asset is his reputation among colleagues and associates. Be suspicious if you do not get straight answers.

> **No credential can guarantee a good surgical result for every patient. There are many factors which contribute to achieving a good surgical result. Probably the most important is the competence of the surgeon.**
>
> **-The American Society For Aesthetic Plastic Surgery**

Walter Erhardt, MD, states, "As more and more Americans choose plastic surgery, the need to check doctors' medical credentials becomes paramount."

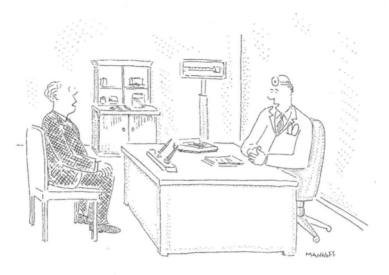

"Hey, how come no diplomas?" "Oh, I'm self-taught."

Information gathering can be confusing, but I will now ease the process for you by listing the four accepted, but minimal, criteria for a surgeon to be considered a recognized specialist in surgery.

1. **Graduation from a recognized school of medicine**

2. **Completion of an ACGME (Accreditation Council for Graduate Medical Education) accredited residency.** The ACGME is composed of representatives of the American Medical Association, the American Board of Medical Specialties, the Association of American Medical Colleges, the Council of Medical Specialty Societies, and the American Hospital Association.

3. **Licensure as a physician and surgeon in the state where he practices**.

4. **Board Certification.** A "board certified" surgeon has met the standard the medical profession accepts as a minimal qualification for one to hold himself to the public and other doctors as a fully trained "specialist." This credential is awarded after successfully completing an approved residency and subsequently mastering a series of written and oral exams. The board may also require practice

experience, and a certain variety of cases performed in that practice for presentation to examiners. Twenty-four medical specialties are represented by a board. In surgery, there are ten boards including orthopedic surgery, eye surgery, chest surgery, neurosurgery, etc. Each specialty's respective board, acting somewhat like a board of directors, is composed of a dozen or so senior members. The board establishes and enforces educational and training requirements for doctors who practice that specialty.

Be advised that the above four training and educational requirements of fully qualified surgeons apply to all recognized surgical specialties. But since cosmetic surgery is not currently an ABMS-sanctioned specialty, you need to know what are the key credentials to look for in the professional bio of one who practices cosmetic surgery. Here is my short checklist:

- **Board certification** in one of the four specialties that legitimately and routinely perform cosmetic procedures within their defined scope of practice: dermatology, head and neck surgery, ophthalmology and plastic surgery.

- **Fellowship training in the cosmetic surgery** of the doctor's board certified specialty.

- **Teaching appointment at a medical school.**

- **Practices exclusively or predominantly cosmetic surgery.**

Consult with a doctor whose professional bio demonstrates these elements and you are in the right pew in the right church.

Other Important Qualifications And Professional Experiences

Following are those credentials, qualifications and professional experiences that I feel are important for the practice of cosmetic surgery.

A qualification considered important is **Fellowship in the American College of Surgeons,** denoted by the initials "FACS" after the doctor's name and MD. Accepted members have met the tests of professional competence and ethics administered by local members of this international society. Only board-certified surgeons are eligible for membership.

You will want to know if your surgeon holds staff membership in accredited hospitals. Although most cosmetic surgery is now performed in office outpatient surgery suites or surgery centers, a hospital staff appointment is always held by conscientious surgeons. In case of emergency or unforeseen events, hospitalization may be necessary. In addition, regular contact between physicians helps keep your doctor abreast of the latest medical advances.

FELLOWSHIP PLEDGE OF THE AMERICAN COLLEGE OF SURGEONS

Recognizing that the American College of Surgeons seeks to exemplify and develop the highest traditions of our profession, I hereby pledge myself as a condition of fellowship in the college, to live in strict accordance with all its principals and regulations. I pledge myself to pursue the practice of surgery with scientific honesty and to place the welfare of my patients above all else; to advance constantly in knowledge; and to render willing help to my collegues, regard their professional interest, and seek their counsel when in doubt as to my own judgement. Upon my honor I hereby declare that I will not practice fee splitting, I further promise to make my fees commensurate with the services rendered and with the patients rights. Moreover, I promise to deal with each patient as I would wish to be dealt with were I in his position. Finally. I pledge myself to cooperate in advancing and extending the ideals and principles of the American College of Surgeons.

Acceptance by his or her professional peers is always important to all high-caliber surgeons. Therefore, *look for membership in county, state and national medical societies.*

> **When one teaches, two learn.**
>
> **-Anonymous**

Many surgeons in private practice hold medical school faculty appointments. Such positions are known as "clinical faculty." Teaching medical students and assisting apprentice surgeons can be a stimulating part of a doctor's professional life. These appointments are part-time and on a voluntary basis without monetary compensation. However, the rewards—including academic stimulation and being at the forefront of medical advances—aren't measured in dollars. Only the most qualified practitioners are honored with such an appointment; therefore, a medical school teaching affiliation is a coveted credential.

Many practicing surgeons own the professional advantage of military service—some of the richest and most practical experience available. *Prior military surgical experience is a huge plus.* A unique, one-time opportunity to sharpen one's professional abilities before entering private practice. I attribute a significant portion of my surgical skills to that early portion of my career.

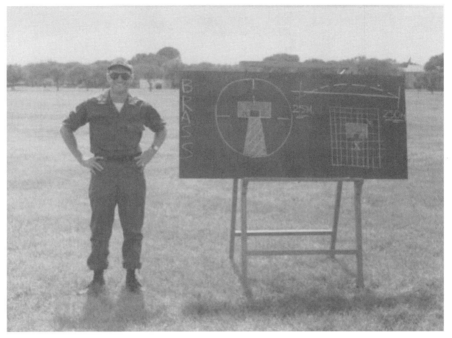

Major R. Kotler, U.S. Army Medical Corps, Fort Sam Houston
Texas, August 1973

Finally, the most critical ingredient of a cosmetic surgeon's training is a fellowship. A fellowship is the highest and most specialized level of professional training and education a physician or surgeon can attain. Such super-focused training is available only after the surgeon has already achieved the status of a fully qualified specialist. Among the surgeons now performing cosmetic surgery, only a small percentage have served cosmetic surgery fellowships. This select group of superspecialists is considered the elite among its peers for having attained this additional, highest-caliber credential.

All his educational and training experiences should be listed in the doctor's professional bio, which should be made available to you. These credentials can be verified by consulting **The Official ABMS** (American Board of Medical Specialties), Directory of Board Certified Medical Specialists, a 581,000 physician profile roster of all board certified specialists. It lists physicians' qualifications, cerification status and biographical information. Available in libraries or can be purchased. The American Board of Medical Specialties also has a public service phone verification hotline: (866) ASK-ABMS.

Four Specialties Legitimately Perform Cosmetic Surgery

Training Differences of the Four Specialties that Perform Cosmetic Surgery			
	General Surgery Residency	Specialty Residency (Minimum Requirement)	Fellowship in Cosmetic Surgery (Optional)
Dermatology		3 years	Full body, skin and related structures
Head & Neck Surgery	1 - 2 years	4 years	Facial only
Ophthalmology		3 years	Eyelids, cheeks, brow
Plastic Surgery	3 - 5 years	2 years	Full body

Depending upon the procedure you desire, surgeons from several different specialties may be qualified and skilled in cosmetic surgery. Which specialties should you expect to encounter during your information gathering?

- **Doctors from various specialties** may refer to themselves as Cosmetic Surgeons. These practitioners usually do not limit themselves to a given region of the body, such as the face and neck. There are no accredited residencies in cosmetic surgery, although fellowships are available to those who have completed residencies in other specialties (such as head and neck surgery or plastic surgery). While an American Board of Cosmetic Surgery exists, it is not recognized by the **American Board of Medical Specialties.**

- **Dermatologists** are skin specialists usually trained in dermabrasion (sanding or planing), chemical and laser peeling for wrinkles and acne, and treatment of spider veins and facial scars. Some dermatologists also perform cosmetic surgery. Certification is granted by the **American Board of Dermatology,** founded in 1932.

Of course, board certification, society memberships, and hospital privileges are just starting points. All they guarantee is that the doctor has the necessary basic training: a medical degree, three years of approved general surgical training, an accredited two- or three-year residency in the specialty, at least two years in practice, and has passed oral and written exams, and has a place to conduct business. Board certification does not guarantee a perfect result.

-Joan Kron, author
Lift: Wanting, Fearing, and Having a Face-Lift

Head and Neck Surgeons are among regional specialists who limit their work to the face and neck. Such surgeons may also perform reconstructive surgery for facial injuries or tumors, but perform no surgery on other parts of the body. Facial plastic (both cosmetic and reconstructive) surgery is a subspecialty of head and neck surgery. The fully qualified head and neck specialist is certified by the **American Board of Otolaryngology**, founded in 1924.

The American Board of Facial Plastic and Reconstructive Surgery. A recent certification process has been developed to recognize specific training in plastic surgery of the face, head, and neck. Surgeons board certified in either plastic surgery or otolaryngology/head and neck surgery are eligible. Requirements are documented training and experience in facial plastic surgery, which may include a one-year fellowship following residency training in a recognized ACGME Otolaryngology or Plastic Surgery program, a minimum two years of practiced experience during which time the surgeon performs a minimum of 100 facial plastic surgery cases and successful completion of a two-day examination.

Hey, if surgery were easy, the janitor could do it.

-David Caldarelli, Jr., MD, supervising me as I struggled through a difficult surgical case as a resident-trainee, at the University of Illinois Medical Center, 1972

The certification recognizes additional capability in facial plastic surgery, including reconstructive and cosmetic procedures. This relatively new board, though not yet recognized by the **American Board of Medical Specialties,** has been deemed equivalent to ABMS boards.

Some eye surgeons, or ophthalmologists, also perform cosmetic surgery on the eyelids and the eyebrows. The **American Board of Facial Plastic Surgery,** founded in 1916, certifies such specialists. Most ophthalmologists who routinely perform cosmetic surgery procedures have served fellowships in ophthalmic plastic surgery.

Policy Statement of the American Medical Association, July 1979

RESOLVED. That it is the American Medical Association policy that individual character, training, comprehension, experience and judgement be the criteria for granting priviledges in hospitals; and

BE IT FURTHER RESOLVED, that physicians representing several specialties can and should be permitted to perform the same procedures if they meet these criteria.

Specialists qualified to perform plastic surgery on all parts of the body are called Plastic Surgeons. Some plastic surgeons focus on breast and body sculpting; others concentrate on the head and neck region; some practice mainly reconstructive surgery, hand surgery or specialize in caring for burn victims through skin grafting. The **American Board of Plastic Surgery**, established in 1937, certifies the qualified specialist.

Specialty Overlap

A confusing issue facing prospective cosmetic surgery patients is specialty overlap: two or more recognized specialties, any of which may be equally capable of performing the same procedure.

INSIDER'S INSIGHT
This Doctor's Ecumenical View
of the Specialty Rivalry

Specialty overlaps spawn specialty rivalry. Head and neck, plastic, ophthalmic plastic, and dermatologic surgeons all have practitioners within their ranks who have a bona fide claim to perform certain cosmetic procedures.

When my patients and my family need cosmetic procedures, I send them to the best doctor— not to a specialty. I refer to the most qualified, talented surgeon I know.

I owe no knee-jerk loyalty to any specialty— even my own. My wife and children have had cosmetic and reconstructive surgery by specialists from all four specialties. Every case was a complete success. Luck? No. Wise choices? Yes!

-RK

As noted previously, four different specialists may perform cosmetic procedures: plastic surgeons, head and neck surgeons, dermatologists and ophthalmologists. Some procedures within each specialty will overlap with some of another specialty. Nasal cosmetic surgery is done by head and neck, or plastic surgeons. Cosmetic surgery of the eyelids and brow is done by plastic surgeons, ophthalmic plastic surgeons (subspecialty-trained ophthalmologists), and head and neck surgeons. Body liposuction, laser, and chemical skin resurfacing are done routinely by some dermatologists, and plastic surgeons.

> **Cosmetic Surgery has a plight of its own. It involves what cosmetic surgeons are and are not, and something needs to be done for the good of patients.**
>
> **-Timothy N. Troy, Editor, Cosmetic Surgery Times**

Not surprisingly, there have been "turf battles" between overlapping specialties. Each of the four specialties lays claim to certain procedures or anatomic regions or "territories." Each has a lobbying arm and public relations experts to protect their "turf" and attract patients. The best course of action for the informed patient is to forget the paid political advertising and follow the common sense, objective, non-partisan roadway laid out in this book.

Hints for Doctor Selection

You must determine if the procedure you are considering is one that the prospective surgeon "majors in." One clever way to determine this is to call the office and ask which five or six procedures the doctor performs most often. If your procedure is not mentioned, you're not talking to the office you want. Move on.

After you have narrowed your search, while visiting doctors' offices, look for the key terms—cosmetic surgery, facial surgery or aesthetic surgery either on business cards, printed material or the office door. These suggest an emphasis on the surgery of appearance vs. general reconstructive surgery. A practice oriented to reconstructive—not cosmetic—surgery could include hand surgery, tumor surgery or treatment of burns. Observe the patients in the waiting room for obvious clues: if most don't seem to be there for cosmetic surgery, you need to, again, move on.

> **INSIDER'S INSIGHT**
>
> Personally, I am always suspicious of arrogant professionals. In my years of dealing with architects, lawyers, accountants, financial specialists, and even dentists and other physicians, I have been happiest with and best served by those without "attitude." There is no reason for airs and posturing by a professional. It only interferes with a productive service.
>
> *-RK*

Hints about the practice's personality also come from décor, and the style, mood, and efficiency of the office. The top professionals surround themselves with *top-notch* staff. Do not be impressed by social column quips, photo opportunities, and fancy offices. Cosmetic surgery is not frivolous. Your appearance is important to you and requires a serious commitment by a surgeon who does not view it as irrelevant or minor. Look for the signs of a perfectionist personality with great seriousness about the work. The surgeon's career spent carrying people's appearance in his hands must be one of complete dedication. Look for a doctor who is positive about cosmetic surgery—someone who is enthusiastic and enjoys all aspects of enhancing your appearance.

A quick, final hint: When comparing surgeons, place their respective professional biographies side by side. The focused cosmetic surgeon's professional history will be replete with references to cosmetic surgery training, experience, research and teaching. A surgeon who does not specialize exclusively in cosmetic surgery may be stronger in other work: cancer, reconstruction, trauma or birth defects. Add this information to what you gather through friends, medical personnel, and the office visit and you will be well on your way to short-listing the best surgeon for your needs.

How Old Should Your Surgeon Be?

Recently, James Sternberg, MD and I were discussing a patient both of us had seen. Dr. Sternberg is a distinguished and senior West Los Angeles dermatologist. I had deep reservations about performing a major face and neck lift because the woman had significant medical problems including liver and lung disease. She was also a heavy smoker—a big red flag. I had called the patient's internist in another city—where she recently lived—and he confirmed her history and endorsed my concern and caution concerning the proposed procedure.

> **Beware of the young doctor and the old barber.**
> -Benjamin Franklin

This woman was adamant about having a facelift. After summarizing my consultation findings, I told her I was uncomfortable and would refuse to operate because of a fear of complications. Dr. Sternberg chuckled and said, "You know, it takes many years of practice before any of us really develops that sixth sense about when to operate and when not to operate, doesn't it?"

That sage comment is the reason for my sharing this story with you. In all medical practices such wisdom, though indefinable, comes very slowly through experience. Indeed anywhere between 10 and 20 years after one starts his practice, the feeling of finally "getting it" arrives.

We are not talking about technical ability here. Manual skills are refined and maximized within a few years of completing one's residency. We are talking about a rite of passage, whereby one outgrows medical adolescence and can rely on a that gut feeling. A doctor's medical "common sense" is continually honed through experience. Gradually, he instinctively knows when to say "yes," "no," or "let's wait."

The seasoned doctor is very comfortable with himself, his skills and his intuition. This security is manifested in confidence in one's abilities and allows a doctor to request a consultation or second opinion before the patient asks. It prompts the surgeon to voluntarily suggest another surgeon who may be more specialized, where it is indicated. A mature practitioner knows what he doesn't know. The real pro has the strength of character and conviction to do the right thing for each patient.

The point is, *chronological age is significant.* Medical education takes decades—college, medical school, internship, residency, fellowship, and finally, practice—all that time to ripen. There is no shortcut to medical maturity.

You do not have to seek the oldest doctor you can find, but consider your own life experience. Are you more skilled at your occupation than you were when you started? After ten or twenty years doing your job, are you better and wiser? There is something to be said for "time on the job" for all of us!

Cosmetic Surgery Ads—Help Or Hype?

STUART and LINCOLN. Attorneys and counselors at law. Will practice jointly in the courts of this judicial circuit. Office no. 4. Hoffman's Row. Upstairs. Springfield.

Advertisement run by two young lawyers, John T. Stuart and Abraham Lincoln. Sangamon Journal, Springfield, Illinois, August 1838.

Advertising is a powerful and pervasive feature of modern American life. Every day, each of us is inundated with radio, television, email, and newspaper and magazine ads. Thousands. Want it or not, they are thrust before us—spaced between what we hear, see, and read.

The practice of cosmetic surgery—like all businesses—has a message to tell about its services. You can investigate further or not. Your choice.

Here is my tip regarding the value of, and your response to, cosmetic surgery ads: *ask yourself if the ad teaches you anything.* I observe two classes of ads: those that educate and those that titillate.

The ads that catch your eye with a busty, voluptuous, no-body-fat, bikini-clad woman probably will not teach you much. The advertiser is attempting to gain your attention with an emotion-only pitch. Some ads catch your eye with lengthy menus of service upon service upon service. But they may gloss over the fact that the surgeon is trying to be all things to all people rather than offer the ideal subspecialty skills patients seek. No education or value here, either.

What I find particularly fascinating about the sexy ad from the "We Do Everything and Anything Cosmetic Surgery Clinic" is that often a doctor's name is not even mentioned. And that may be because these clinics are often owned by businessmen who hire doctors as contractors. That is not generally the best way for physicians to practice medicine. They are not invested, figuratively and literally, in the practice and the standards therefore can be a bit irregular. And humorously, since California, at least, requires truth in advertising and insists that the featured voluptuous female be identified as either a patient or not a patient, most of these high profile clinics are apparently unable to produce even one excellent result worthy of being included in the ad. The caption below the young lady's photograph invariably states "model." Why would anyone ever go to a clinic that cannot even show off a single credible result?

> **INSIDER'S INSIGHT**
>
> Look closely at advertisements, particularly ones that feature a pretty, shapely lady, not a patient but a model. A patient photo might inspire more confidence —so would a doctor's name and credentials.
>
> *-RK*

The alternative is an ad that teaches and enlightens you, as does a good book. The high quality ad tells a story: perhaps a patient shares his or her experience with cosmetic surgery, or serial ads may explain common cosmetic surgery procedures. Such ads make you smarter. They are more sophisticated and will appeal to the thoughtful person who is conducting a rational—and not purely emotional—search for cosmetic surgery services. And, yes, these ads can inform and educate, even without the glitzy artwork or photos!

Two more thoughts for your consideration. Some folks have an inherent distrust of professionals who advertise—not just cosmetic surgeons—but lawyers, accountants, financial advisers, etc. Their knee-jerk response, when asked why, is:

● "How good can they be if they advertise?"

● "Don't they get enough clients (or patients) through referral, without advertising?"

● "High quality professionals and companies don't advertise. They don't have to. Everybody knows they're good."

Contending that quality professionals do not advertise is incorrect. For example, one of the attorneys I've used for years—a superspecialist, I might add—came to my attention through an informative ad in our county medical association newsletter. His advertisement was an education in print. I immediately learned that his specialty practice matched my need. He has done excellent work, at very reasonable fees for me, for twenty years. If I hadn't seen his ad, I might never have benefited from his expertise!

To those who fret that professionals who advertise need the ad power to keep them busy, I ask: What is wrong with being busy? When I want surgery, I will be happy to hear that my surgeon has a full schedule; you cannot maintain your surgical skills as "an occasional operator." I like to patronize busy professionals; they are focused and they are at the top of their game. The more they perform their work, the better their work is.

Finally, there are the *hoity toities* who snobbishly sneer at advertising by professionals. They contend that top-quality practitioners and businesses are so well known that their reputations obviate the need to advertise. For them following question: If you drive a Mercedes or buy that special gift at Cartier or Tiffany, might your patronage have been motivated by an advertisement?

Yes, Cartier, Tiffany, Mercedes, and even Rolls Royce, advertise. Established companies selling quality products know the value of their products, and recognize the value of advertising them to an ever-widening audience. You just might want to amend any negative feelings by realizing that professionals who provide top quality services, including cosmetic surgeons, want to teach and enlighten you. And they want to tell you why they are special and valuable. Just like Lexus, Nordstrom and IBM.

I rest my case.

An attractive young woman was being shown around the ship by Tim, a young intern. "And what is your specialty?" asked the woman.

"I'm a naval surgeon," Tim responded.

"My oh, my," sighed the woman. "Medicine is certainly getting specialized these days!"

-Sid Behrman
The Doctor's Joke Book

4

WHY SUPERSPECIALIZATION Is So IMPORTANT

Secret: The doctor you want is called a *superspecialist*— he practices cosmetic surgery exclusively.

IT'S EASY TO APPRECIATE THE VALUE OF NARROW SPECIALIZATION. Our society lives in a time of increasing specialization in all endeavors. Professionals in every line of work exemplify this trend. A football tackle would probably make a lousy quarterback, a position that requires a different mindset and other skills. The classical violinist seldom features bluegrass as part of his repertoire. Would you hire an electrical engineer or a chemical engineer to build a highway?

PATIENT COMMENT

Dear Dr. Kotler:

Like yourself, I am a physician. I direct a national referral center in Ann Arbor, Michigan. My patients come from throughout the world, as do yours, and suffer from severe and painful conditions. Many of our patients have obstructive nasal deformities. Some require functional reconstruction and cosmetic attention to the deformity. Your work had been known to me for years, and I elected to send several individuals to you for necessary surgery.

I am writing to tell you that I am delighted with the results. In addition to relieving symptoms, you were able to achieve an incredibly natural look. These individuals do not look as though they have had reconstructive surgery. More specifically, they do not look as though they have "someone else's" face or nose. They are pleased, and so am I.

As medicine has become more complex, there is a need for advanced training, even within the specialties. Super-specialization seems to be a trend that is unavoidable. A need to acquire more knowledge and greater technical skills has mandated this change. The work you have done on those I have sent you illustrates the benefit of your superspecial-ization. Congratulations.

Sincerely,
Joel R. Saper, MD, FACP, FAAN
Founder and Director of
Michigan Head Pain & Neurological Institute
Ann Arbor, MI

In surgery, as in many disciplines, the best results are realized when a team of highly skilled individuals perform the same procedure(s) on a daily basis. Not unlike a soccer team or an orchestra. Repetition makes for perfection. In this instance, the team is built around the surgeon. So, selecting the most highly specialized surgeon to lead the team is the single most important step in achieving satisfaction from cosmetic surgery.

Plastic surgery now has so many subspecialties, it is impossible for anyone to do everything equally well.

-Robert Goldwyn, MD
Harvard University
Medical School
author, *Beyond Appearance:*
Reflections of a Plastic
Surgeon

Therefore, it is imperative that prospective patients find a specialist whose exclusive, or major, concentration is cosmetic surgery, with particular expertise in the specific procedure desired.

Today, because of the evolution to narrow specialization and sophistication, it is impossible to be a successful "jack of all trades." Plastic surgery of the body—cosmetic and reconstructive—is far too broad and complex for any one doctor to master. Similarily, in the surgical world, focus on a given region of the body has been the trend: hand surgery, foot surgery, chest surgery, and eye surgery. Such specialization has narrowed even further via subspecialization. Now, there are eye surgeons who limit their practice to the retina and chest surgeons who perform only open-heart procedures.

The fine honing of specialization in modern medical practice is known as *superspecialization:* a narrow, focused, "boutique" practice. Great benefits to the patient are realized when a surgeon narrows his scope and concentrates on a limited selection of procedures.

The patient's question might now become, "How do I differentiate between specialist, subspecialist, and superspecialist?" The following graphic, The **Hierarchy of Modern Medical Superspecialization** will help you understand the medical profession's stratification. The same applies to all specialties; some internists subspecialize in endocrinology; then a limited number of endocrinologists superspecialize in thyroid disorders only.

The pyramid narrows as specialization narrows. The number of practitioners decreases commensurate with the further specialization.

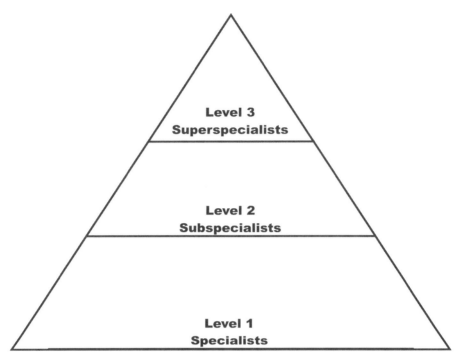

The Hierarchy of Modern Medical Superspecialization

Cosmetic Surgery Hierarchy

Level 1:   *Specialist.* Some cosmetic surgery but most time spent on reconstructive surgery for disease or accident. Board certified. No fellowship training.

Level 2:   *Subspecialist.* Practices both reconstructive and cosmetic procedures, but not the full scope of the parent specialty. Typically board certified plus fellowship training beyond his residency.

Level 3:   *Superspecialist.* Practices cosmetic surgery exclusively. No reconstructive surgery. Typically board certified and fellowship trained, the most specialized of all practitioners. In the world of cosmetic surgery, these doctors are at the apex of sophistication, training, and skill.

> We live in an age when medical and scientific progress is unfolding at such an enormously rapid pace that it is difficult for one individual to keep track of, let alone master, developments in even a small area of medicine.
>
> -Kurt J. Wagner, MD, Gerald Imber, MD, authors, *Beauty By Design*

You read in **Chapter 3** about board certification. The board awards a certificate or diploma to successful applicants signifying the new doc has met all the board's prescribed standards. He is now considered a qualified specialist in the eyes of the specialty and the medical profession has met all the board's prescribed standards. He is now considered a qualified specialist in the eyes of the specialty and the medical profession.

Because residency is such an intense and concentrated period of study and experience, the young specialist, who just passed his exams, will never be more knowledgeable about the entire spectrum of that specialty. The brains of those "just out of training" are brimming with encyclopedic textbook and medical journal knowledge.

Armed with much theoretical knowledge but little or no clinical (practice) experience, the young surgeon is, nonetheless, qualified to open his own practice. But for a few there may come an awakening of sorts. Acknowledging that medical knowledge is expanding rapidly, doubling every ten years, there comes a concern: "I am not sure I can do this entire specialty and do it all well. My specialty is too broad." That introspective, objective, and ethical doctor-specialist realizes that to be competent, he must focus on just one aspect of his practice. At the same time, he must continue to learn more techniques and skills. This is known as subspecialization or regional specialization.

> One finds one's life evolving and interests evolving, and the more I became acquainted with aesthetic (cosmetic) surgery, I recognized that it was far more challenging. There was much less (tolerance for making) an error in aesthetic surgery than in reconstructive procedures.
>
> - John Grossman, MD Interview, *Cosmetic Surgery Times*

You see examples of this in orthopedic surgery, another specialty servicing the body from head to toe. It has developed well-defined subspecialties to maximize the practioner's effectiveness and to improve surgical results for the patient. Orthopedists may subspecialize in joint replacement, spine surgery or sports medicine. Orthopedic's superspecialists include knee surgeons and hand surgeons.

Ophthalmology, the oldest medical specialty, long ago divided itself into recognized subspecialties even though the eye and auxiliary structures occupy only a few cubic inches of the body: surgery of the retina, corneal surgery, plastic surgery of the eyelids and orbits, and pediatric ophthalmology.

> **Ophthalmology is a field that is characterized by subspecialization. Comprehensive ophthalmologists (generalists who do not focus their practice on an ophthalmic subspecialty) continue to represent the majority of practicing ophthalmologists. Nationally, one-fourth of graduating ophthalmology residents go on to fellowship training, and at academic programs, it is not unusual for the majority of the graduating class to pursue subspecialty fellowship training. Especially in urban areas, ophthalmic subspecialties often limit their practice to their subspecialty and do not take care of general problems such as cataracts.**
>
> **Even within the ophthalmic subspecialties, there is a tendency for further specialization. For example, some cornea fellowships and cornea specialists focus exclusively on refractive surgery (LASIK is an example of refractive surgery). Orbital, facial, and ophthalmic plastic surgery is a broad discipline and there has been a tendency towards additional specialization in aesthetic (cosmetic) surgery, lacrimal (tear duct) surgery, and orbital surgery.**
>
> **Oculoplastic surgery is a relatively young subspecialty.... The field has exploded... and is evolving into a broader discipline. There are now more than 400 members of the American Society of Ophthalmic Plastic and Reconstructive Surgery. Fellowships are two years long with many fellows taking additional subspecialty training after two years of fellowship.**
>
> **– Norman Shorr, MD, FACS,**
> **Robert Alan Goldberg, MD, FACS and Todd Cook, MD**
> **"What's New in Ophthalmic Plastic Surgery,"**
> *Journal of the American College of Surgeons,*
> **November 2001**

Within plastic surgery you can find subspecialty surgeons concentrating on cosmetics, pediatrics, head and neck, cancer, burns, hands, etc. One of modern plastic surgery's greatest accomplishments has been the development and evolution of craniofacial surgery, the challenging, complicated, multi-stage repair of birth defects and rebuilding of the skull and face. A select number of plastic surgeons limit their practice to this young and very narrow superspecialty.

The importance of fellowships cannot be underestimated. The refinement and focus of subspecialty education will continue to narrow as we recognize that to achieve surgical excellence it requires depth of knowledge that is more valuable than width.

> **The science of surgery becomes more complex and demanding daily, such that only the specialist can hope to be current and capable and expert in the limited field.**
>
> **-Loring W. Pratt, MD Former Regent, American College of Surgeons**

> **It's known that surgeons who do large numbers of a procedure get very good at that procedure.**
>
> **-Lloyd Nyhus, MD Profession of Surgery, University of Illinois College of Medicine, Chicago**

Typically, subspecialty fellowships are developed and monitored by specialty or subspecialty societies. They are not directly governed by the boards of the parent specialties. The American Academy of Dermatology, the continuing education arm of that specialty, oversees fellowships in skin cancer surgery and pediatric dermatology. The American Academy of Facial Plastic and Reconstructive Surgery provides fellowship opportunities in cosmetic and reconstructive surgery of the face, head and neck. The American Society of Plastic Surgeons offers fellowships in head and neck tumor surgery, pediatric surgery, and full body cosmetic surgery.

By now you should have no doubt that the more specialized the doctor, the greater likelihood of good results for you, the patient. You now know that if you are considering a facelift, you should seek a board certified specialist who focuses on cosmetic surgery and ideally has done a cosmetic surgery fellowship. A cosmetic surgery superspecialist will typically limit his practice to fifteen or fewer procedures mastered after lifelong study, focus and dedication.

A Short History of Superspecialization

The history of surgery is one of continual progress made through deliberate narrowing and specialization by surgical practitioners. Only 85 years ago, there were no specialties within surgery itself. All surgery, from brain to toe, was done by "a surgeon." And at that time, the "surgeon" had no formal specialty training after completion of medical school. But the trend today in medical education is to train doctors who will be more skillful in a relatively limited portion of the body. A "jack of all trades" and, hence, "master of none" is not satisfactory in today's highly specialized medical world. This is why, even within a recognized specialty such as plastic surgery, there are great benefits to the public when a surgeon narrows his scope choosing not to perform most other operations within the broad specialty.

How Changes In Medical Education Encourage Superspecialization

I would like to share with you the reasons why I chose to limit my practice to cosmetic surgery of the face and neck, exclusively. It was a very important decision.

> Let us be thankful that the day of the all-around surgical specialist is done! Surgery is not advanced by that type of activity… no matter how talented the surgeon, he cannot do equally as good work in all of these provinces.
>
> -Owen H. Wangensteen, MD
> Professor of Surgery,
> University of Minnesota
> in a paper delivered before the
> American College of Surgeons

Over 35 years ago, in the mid-60s, as a medical student, it became obvious to me that modern medicine was expanding and improving very quickly, primarily because of specialization. Hand surgery, burn surgery, heart surgery, artery and vein surgery were beginning to be separated from their parent subspecialties. These and others were being practiced as distinct specialties. Later, I realized that if I were to excel at my chosen work, I would have to be as specialized as possible. It was easily recognizable that the

> In today's supertrained society, the finest and most rigidly prepared specialists are readily available.
>
> - Kurt J. Wagner, MD, and Gerald Imber, MD
> *Beauty by Design*

more specialized the doctor, the greater the likelihood of good results for the patient. Therefore, my decision to pursue a course of education and training would allow me to bring the highest degree of skill to my patients. I wanted to excel in the performance of just a few procedures. In short, I wanted to be a *superspecialist* because it would be better for my patients. That meant ultimately limiting my practice to six or fewer procedures within a specific region of the body.

A Personal Decision is Made

Since I enjoyed the face and neck work most, I elected to forego "training in body surgery." No hand surgery, no breast or body sculpturing. No treatment of burns. No correction of birth defects or major body cancer surgery. While these surgical services were important, other colleagues would choose to specialize in those.

As my plan evolved, I felt it was best not to perform accident or emergency room work any longer. They would detract from my devotion to those elective scheduled procedures that I preferred. I didn't want to be up all night in an emergency room sewing up an accident victim and not be well rested for someone's facelift the next morning. I would be left to do what I enjoyed doing most—improving people's appearance.

In summary, as I kiddingly tell my patients: "I am sorry but we don't do body and fender work, but we have excellent associates who do." Patients do understand, instinctively, the importance of choosing a doctor whose focus matches their specific need. Now, with increasing frequency, we hear patients say: "I want a cosmetic surgeon who doesn't *do everything*." The public has endorsed superspecialization by increasingly patronizing the more specialized and focused doctors.

Patients Now Seek The Most Specialized

So, patients "get it." They sense, intuitively, that a "super-specialist" is more likely to perform—for them—at the highest level, rather than the "I do everything" doctor. That mastery comes only with focus, dedication and long study. No different than that required for greatness by a piano virtuoso or a football place kicker. As one patient commented: "Since you have choices—and time to do research—why would anyone not use the most specialized cosmetic surgeon?"

Having practiced in my community for over 25 years, I'm familiar with colleagues who are as specialized in their work as I am in mine. Patients are entitled to a referral to the most highly qualified consultants. There should only be one concern: what is best, not for the doctor, but for the patient. Superspecialization achieves that end. Insist on it for yourself.

Top Athletes Are One-Sport Superspecialists

Michael Jordan, the basketball wonder, had a one year baseball career. An adequate outfielder, he hit .202 in 127 games, striking out 114 times in 436 at bats. Jordan belted 3 home runs, collected 51 RBIs, and stole 30 bases. He also led all Southern League outfielders with 11 errors.

-courtesy Lee Kotler, former sportswriter, *Chicago Tribune*

INSIDER'S INSIGHT

Why Cosmetic Surgery Superspecialists Congregate in Certain Larger Cities

Every American can readily identify artistic centers of excellence where superior skills and talent congregate. Nashville for country and western music; for major theater, the Big Apple — New York City. Our best jazz? New Orleans or Memphis.

Where then would you expect to find the top country's cosmetic surgery superspecialists? The flocking of these surgical artists is driven by population and the local cultures' fashion consciousness. Many such practitioners gather in New York City and Los Angeles because each city is a commercial, cultural and professional hub for a region of over 14 million people. The patient pool is huge. So, you won't find the same corps of talent in Small Town, USA because the patient pool is relatively small. Plus, certain regions of the U.S. have greater numbers of style and appearance aficionados. Label them trendier. Documented by statistics, their inhabitants also have a greater taste for cosmetic surgery and its allied services.

The populations of the Northeast, Southern California, and the tip of Florida – the coastals — are much more into matters of appearance. But why there? It's not the water. No, it's because these are homes to our fashion and entertainment industries. Beauty is big. Not that looking good is universally frowned upon elsewhere. But, by contrast, in the Midwest heartland, in the rugged Pacific Northwest, and in our last frontier—the Southwest—the quest for youth and the search for the ideal face and body rank lower on personal agendas. Not absent from the to-do list, just a few lines down.

Clustering of high level practitioners is always good news for patients. The naturally-occurring competition between these heavyweights doing big volumes of cosmetic surgery raises the performance bar to the highest level. To mastery, not just competence. Better results —fewer disappointments. Mediocrity gets crowded out. Those occasional cosmetic surgeons, operating in a low-demand climate, rarely cut it. Without an active case load, the skill level stagnates. That's why locales with little appetite for cosmetic surgery will never attract the top superspecialists.

-RK

Never go to a doctor whose plants have died.
-Erma Bombeck in *The Doctor Joke Book*

5

The CONSULTATION

Secret: Many consultations focus on selling, not teaching. When is a "free" consultation too expensive?

WHEN HAVE YOU EVER PAID TO HEAR A SALESPERSON'S PRESENTATION? Probably never. In the world of cosmetic surgery, the "free consultation" is usually conducted not by the physician who would be your surgeon but by a professional salesperson. Dubbed "consultant," they often work on commission. Many cosmetic surgery practices are high-volume, clinic-type enterprises where the business strategy is to process as many prospective patients as possible. Since the doctor cannot possibly deal with the demand for "free" consults by himself, the *consultant/ salesperson* takes over that function. It is a necessary "sorting out" process. This being the case, "free" is just the right price.

> Doctors usually charge a consultation fee for your first visit, which may be as much as $150 or more (applied against your surgery fees), but the amount of their initial consultation fee should not really play a role in deciding with whom you consult. After all, you will presumably be spending thousands of dollars on surgery which costs many more thousands to try to correct elsewhere if done poorly, so an extra $200-$300 in consultation fees should not be the basis for narrowing the field. I thought I was saving money by consulting with six doctors who charged no initial fee, but in hindsight, I realized that the best doctor was the seventh one who charged a $75 fee (he ended up correcting part of my botched surgery). I feel that doctors who charge no consultation fee use it as a sales tool to attract clients while those who charge a fee may be relying more on their reputations.
>
> - Mark Sugar, author
> *A Guide to Choosing a Good Plastic Surgeon*

The Ideal Cosmetic Surgery Consultation
Is an Examination *of the Doctor!*

Think of this book as a study guide. It leads you through the consultation course. It opens your eyes and tunes up your ears. It gives you the vocabulary of the cosmetic surgery world: procedure names in both English and medicalese. So you can speak the same language as the lady or gentleman in the white coat. You're crossing the border into another country, but you will speak the language.

> **The best candidate for surgery is someone who has realistic expectations of what can be attained with her own anatomy (and age). That applies to everything from a face lift to breast augmentation.**
>
> **-Sherrell J. Aston, MD,**
> ***Allure*, March 2001**

This book will serve you best when under-lined, highlighted and crammed with margin notes. Hopefully, it will even be dog-eared because you wisely read and reread it. It is just like school, again. But now, it is not learning for learning's sake or for A's and B's to raise your grade point. You want to learn so your consultation is valuable to you. Think of the consultation as an exam. But an open book exam. You open the book, start asking really sharp questions, and the examination of the doctor has begun.

Although we instinctively respond to "free" products and services of any type, you must be skeptical when you sense this marketing tactic applied to medical procedures. When consulting for such an important professional service as a face lift, you need time with the doctor—not a salesperson. And "time" is the critical issue. A doctor's time may cost you something, but **only the doctor can help you assess risk and decide on the type of procedure(s)** necessary to achieve the results you seek. Only the doctor can say "go" or "no go."

First Contact—Early Clue About An Office's Quality

One barometer of an office's quality is how your first phone call is handled. Doesn't that make sense? Hasn't your experience given you clues about whether or not you want to do business with certain companies strictly based on how they handled your inquiry?

When I call a professional office, within the first twenty seconds, I can sense whether or not I am speaking with a high-quality, service-oriented, sharp practice. Here are my criteria for excellence:

● The call is answered after no more than four rings.

- You should never get a busy signal.

- You are greeted by a warm, courteous, cheery, glad-to-be-of-service staff member. You can almost see the smile through the telephone line.

- The person answering your call is knowledgeable, helpful, and able to answer most or all questions promptly. You sense that she has been well trained to help and educate you. What you don't want to hear is, "Gee, I don't know," with the conversation dropped right there.

- If there is a question she cannot answer, you are promptly transferred to another staff member who is qualified and who can answer it.

- You are offered additional, complementary teaching aids, e.g., brochures, pamphlets, video- or audiotapes, etc. These further explain the services available to you. And, they will be U.S. mailed, emailed, or faxed promptly. Most surgeons provide prospective patients with appropriate brochures and pamphlets prior to the consultation. This allows the patient to review important points about the procedure(s) under consideration. Being prepared in advance guarantees a more productive session with the doctor. Questions raised while reading this material can be specifically answered during the consultation.

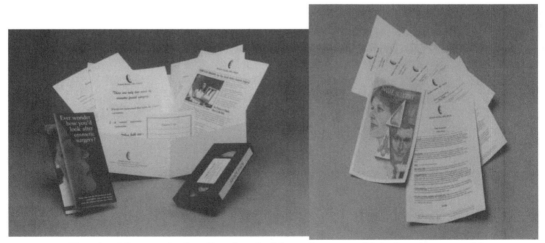

You should request educational materials such as pamphlets, brochures or videos before you consult. You will better prepared and will maximize your time with doctor and staff.

- If you decide to schedule a consultation, you are offered several choices for your convenience.

- The day, date and time are confirmed with you prior to the conversation's end. You are also assured that you will receive a written confirmation including directions to the office and parking advice.

- As the conversation ends, you are reminded of the name or names of the staff members with whom you spoke. You are encouraged to call them if you have any further questions. These are your "contact" people.

- If you ask about fees, you receive some meaningful information. While an exact fee quotation requires a consultation and evaluation by the doctor, a superior office will offer a "range of fees" or "most common fee" for the procedure or procedures you are interested in. You have the right to know so you can evaluate whether your budget is "within the ballpark."

- Finally, the office will ask for your daytime and evening phone numbers so you can be contacted several days prior to your consultation. They will want to be certain you received the promised information and also confirm the appointment particulars. Having your phone numbers also allows the office to inform you should any change in the office's schedule affect your appointment time.

Is all this important? I think so. Consider yourself a customer. Want good service? Service begins with that first telephone call. Every practice takes its cues from the top; the doctor sets the standards; it is his practice; he is the boss.

The doctor must care about you, the caller, before he ever meets you. If not, if he does not have in place smart, able, and conscientious staff "up front," how particular, how attentive, and how competent might he and his team be in the operating room and during the recovery phase? Think about it.

Now you know how to sort cosmetic surgeons within five minutes for just the price of a phone call.

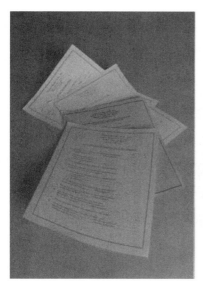

You will most likely be asked to fill out questionaires.

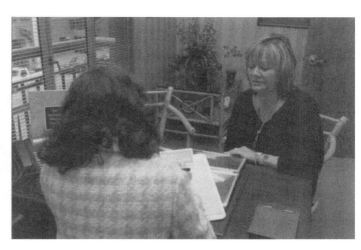

Your consultation begins with your medical history.

Getting The Best from Your Doctor and His Staff

The Consultation

Karel Rall, Patient Counselor at the Cosmetic Surgery Specialists Medical Group of Beverly Hills, tells us that the best care will be the happy result of a partnership between you and your doctor and his staff. Here's how to achieve that partnership:

● **When you schedule your consultation, be as specific as you can about your desires.** For example, if you are consulting because you had an unsuccessful nasal surgery previously, please tell the staff member that. Why? Because that will trigger some responses from them that can optimize the value of your consultation, and make it more efficient. Hearing that you wish to discuss a possible second surgery, you will be advised to bring copies of your medical records and photographs from your first surgery (you can get them easily by calling or writing to your previous surgeon's office). Having all your records will help the consulting doctor give his best recommendation at your first meeting.

● **You will get more out of the consultation by preparing for it.** Study the educational materials the doctor has sent you in response to your initial call for information. Write down the questions you wish to ask.

● **Bring a friend or relative with you.** "Four ears and four eyes are twice as good for learning." Your companion may see or hear something that you may miss. The idea is to leave the consultation armed with as much information as possible.

● **Take notes.** Write down the responses/answers to your listed questions. Then you can review them at home. Compare the answers to the same questions posed to different doctors.

● **Use Dr. Kotler's checklist** in Appendix D, page 248. It makes the information gathered at several consultations easier to evaluate.

When you arrive for your consultation, you should be warmly greeted by a friendly staff that is sincere, efficient and helpful. Surgical practice is comprised of more than the services of your surgeon. A good surgeon surrounds himself with a strong team to support his efforts. Members of that team are an extension of the surgeon. Their professionalism and attentiveness should mirror his. The staff may help obtain your complete health history and answer general questions. The environment should be comfortable. You should feel "at home."

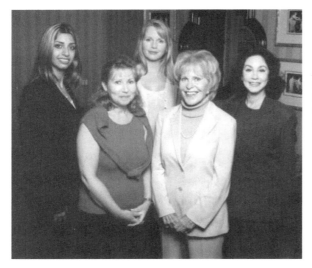

A friendly staff always adds to the quality of your experience before and after surgery. They should make you feel at home.

Photographs of you will be taken sometime during the consultation visit. Keep in mind these pictures are not glamour shots. They are not intended to be flattering nor are they for public view. High-resolution medical photographs showing every wrinkle, crease or bulge must be studied and reviewed by the surgeon in preparation for your operation, and will be consulted during your procedure as well. They are essential blueprints for the surgeon.

> **It is just as important for the doctor to know what you like about yourself as what you want to change.**
>
> -Nola Rocco, author
> *A Facelift Is a Bargain*

The interview with the surgeon should be relaxed, enjoyable and informative. The competent doctor wants to learn your specific desires so he can determine the practicality of the surgery you request. He must be confident that your expectations are realistic and can be met. Your medical history will be reviewed and you should be carefully examined. Specific procedures should be discussed in detail and in nonmedical terms. Your questions should be answered with frankness and patience. It is important to note that not everyone is a good candidate for cosmetic surgery. The main goal of the consultation is to determine if it is the right thing for you. The doctor's recommendation might be to do nothing!

WHO KNOWS BEST?

When it comes to deciding what you should or should not have done, *you do*, insists John E. Sherman, MD, New York City. 'When patients are dissatisfied, it's often because they underwent surgery that they never wanted in the first place.' That can be due to pressure from friends and family, or surgeons who push patients into procedures they never would have considered otherwise. Still, you have to balance that with the benefits of an informed consultation, notes Dr. Sherman. 'You may come in saying you want eyelid surgery when your real problem could be solved with a brow lift.' You and your doctor should be able to come to a mutually agreeable conclusion. If you walk in thinking you would like a facelift and the surgeon tries to sell you a head-to-toe liposuction, you are not on the same wavelength and you should go elsewhere. You want to work with someone who has your best interests at heart, and your priorities in mind.

-M. Katherine Francis, author
"A Guide to Plastic Surgery—
An All You Need To Know Primer for First Timers,"
Longevity magazine

You and your doctor must spend time getting to know each other. If you need more time—and that happens frequently—the doctor should welcome you back for one or more "re-consultations." The time you spend upfront—before the operation—is your most valuable.

Remember, Cosmetic Surgery Is Only for the Healthy

In our practice, my staff is probably tired of hearing my mantra: "We don't take chances." That's what business people call "risk management." And the most significant risk reducer for a patient is being in tip-top physical condition. Our practice has an inviolate rule that a complete physical examination is done several weeks prior to the surgical procedure. We ask that the patient's personal physician perform the examination and review the cardiogram and laboratory tests we request. Our vigilance in this "last stop before surgery" is essential because an unrecognized medical condition could have a bearing on the safety of the anesthetic, and even the result of the operation.

My advice: "Assume nothing." Even though you feel well, unless you've had a complete physical examination within thirty days prior to your scheduled procedure, it is essential to have your personal doctor perform one. We insist on it; so should your surgeon. Cosmetic surgery, never an emergency, can wait. When you go forward, it must be under ideal circumstances. *Don't take chances.*

INSIDER'S INSIGHT

Several years ago, our usual, requisite and preoperative examina-tion revealed a significant anemia (low red blood cell count). Surgery was cancelled. It was determined quickly that the low blood count was due to internal bleeding, from the colon, indi-cating an early, small cancer. The patient –unaware of this potentially serious medical problem–was deeply appreciative of our cautious approach that led to an unan-ticipated discovery. She wrote: "Your completeness in preparation for surgery is so wise, and in my case, life saving".

-RK

PATIENT COMMENTARY

As a doctor, your attentiveness before and after the surgery, was so very reassuring and most appreciated. Your staff should also be commended. I can't tell you how many offices I had been to where staff members tried to bully me into scheduling the procedure, where the doctor was far too busy to answer my questions personally, and one of the doctors

> *was just plain arrogant. You and your staff were concerned about my health and me and were always informative, prompt and helpful.*
>
> *-Heidi, student*

The 15 Smartest Questions to Ask Your Prospective Surgeon

Secret: **Unique Insider Information. A shortcut to sort out the most qualified doctors.**

Asking questions is an art form. Conducting an interview is a learned skill. It is difficult for many people to construct an analytical approach when consulting with professionals. It is particularly challenging in the world of cosmetic surgery—where emotion can override wisdom. Following are 15 powerful questions to keep you on track:

1. Do you practice cosmetic surgery exclusively? What percentage is performed on the face? What percentage is performed on other parts of the body?

2. If you don't perform cosmetic surgery exclusively, what percentage of the practice is dedicated to cosmetic vs. reconstructive surgery?

3. How long have you been performing the procedures I am considering? How many of these procedures do you perform in a year?

4. Do you have hospital privileges to perform the procedures I am requesting?

5. Did you serve a fellowship in cosmetic surgery? If fellowship trained, how long was the fellowship? What types of cases did you perform, assist in or observe during your fellowship?

6. Have you written books or authored journal articles on facial cosmetic surgery? On body cosmetic surgery?

7. Do you teach other doctors your techniques of cosmetic surgery?

8. May I receive a copy of your professional biography summarizing your training, qualifications and credentials to perform the procedures I want?

9. Can I speak to a patient who's had a similar procedure performed by you?

10. Where is the surgery to take place? Your office? Outpatient surgery center? Hospital? Whichever it is, is it licensed by the state and /or the U.S. government? Or is it accredited by The Joint Commission on Accreditation of Ambulatory Health Organizations or by The Accreditation Association for Ambulatory Health Care or The American Association for Accreditation of Ambulatory Surgical Facilities?

11. Will I need to have a physical examination and lab tests prior to surgery? Who does this—you, or my primary physician?

12. What type of anesthesia can I expect? Local anesthesia only, local anesthesia with sedation or general anesthesia? Why do you choose that type? Who will administer the anesthetic? A doctor anesthesiologist, a nurse anesthetist, or you? How long will I be "under"?

13. What are the most common complications of this procedure? Which is the most serious? How would these be anticipated and/or corrected?

14. What if I need a redo or touchup procedure? Will there be additional charges by the surgeon? By the surgery center? By the anesthesiologist?

15. What stages of healing can I expect? How long are each of these? When can I resume my daily activities? What follow up can I expect from you and your office?

A wise man is one who never asks a question he doesn't know the answer to...before he buys. He knows what the "right answer" should be. Many surgeons could answer the questions above. How can you be sure the answer you get is the right one? Be wise. Know the answers you are looking for. By the time you turn the last page of this book, you will recognize the correct answer when you hear it.

COMPUTER IMAGING

Secret: A consultation without computer imaging has limited value. You need to see on a computer screen what you will look like "after."

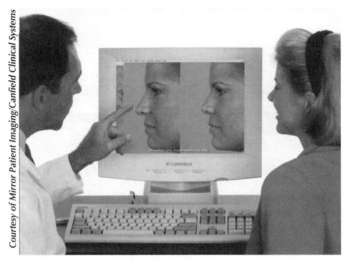

Courtesy of Mirror Patient Imaging/Canfield Clinical Systems

See your predicted result on a computer screen.

"Doctor, what will I look like after surgery?" While it cannot predict final results with 100 percent accuracy, computer imaging is unquestionably the best technique available today to help you clearly understand what the doctor can—or cannot—do for you. Once you are clear on the procedures, or combination of procedures, computer imaging is a must! A computer screen becomes your personal crystal ball and will graphically demonstrate what you can expect.

During a computer imaging session, a standard video camera captures two identical photos of your face or body and freezes them onto a computer screen. The image on the left is the unchanged "before." The right hand image becomes the "after," as the doctor or assistant changes the shape of the nose or removes eyelid bags through the use of a computer "pen." Comparing the predicted "after" to the "before", allows you to see what cosmetic surgery can or cannot do for you. You deserve to utilize the latest technology allowing you to visualize the surgeon's proposal. Computer imaging is a fantastic communication tool that affords a "meeting of the minds." A consultation without it has limited value.

PATIENT COMMENTARY

> *Pearl was especially helpful with her computer skills and patience as she worked with me to find the right "after" image. Consulting with surgeons for cosmetic facial surgery is not an easy task, but you made it much easier by providing this tool to help establish clear communication. The fact that you offer access to this service through the Internet is convenient for anyone considering this type of surgery.*
>
> *-Richard, graphic artist, California*

Reviewing the "Before" and "After" Album
A Procedural Guide

Secret: A surgeon's "before" and "after" album is filled with clues. You should see lots of photos—and they must be photographically "honest."

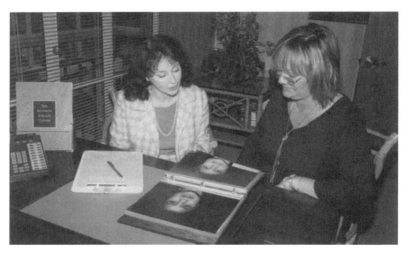

Viewing Before & After Albums.

The purpose of the consultation with the cosmetic surgeon is to learn more. One of the most valuable components of that visit is the chance to view a large number of typical "before and after" examples. A primary reason for post surgical remorse is failure to study the doctor's work. You need to get a sense of his art form, his style, and his results. These photographs offer an impression of that particular

> **Choose your surgeon carefully; check him out before you check out, and then look at before and after pictures of his patients. The after pictures should look better.**
>
> -Joan Rivers

surgeon's idea of reasonable improvement. They also help give you, the patient, a grasp of the realistic results of cosmetic surgery.

I'm often amazed when I learn of people who have been disappointed with their cosmetic surgery and when asked: "Did you see the doctor's work before?" they state, "No. I asked to see before and after pictures at the consultation but the doctor didn't have any." What nonsense!

If you see consistent evidence of substantial, yet natural change in appearance, you will probably be comfortable in that surgeon's hands. If the results look artificial, unnatural, overdone or in any way displeasing, your taste may be better served by another doctor. Remember you are seeking natural—not "plastic"—surgery. And, you want to look better—not different.

An Important Commentary Regarding Medical Photography

Here are important comments on medical photography by David J. Terris, MD, Associate Professor, Head and Neck Surgery, Stanford University, as stated in the October, 2001, issue of *Cosmetic Surgery Times*, a news journal for cosmetic surgeons. Dr. Terris' remarks are directed to cosmetic surgeons' presentations—to their colleagues—at medical meetings, seminars, and in medical papers. However, this commentary is equally appropriate to understand the importance of photographic consistency and honesty in the doctor's before and after photo collection:

"It's usually not a situation where an investigator is deliberately trying to alter results or mislead the audience. But through inadvertently changing the techniques that they use preoperatively to postoperatively, they can make it difficult to compare appearances before and after procedures." Dr. Terris then stated: "Such researchers mislead not only their audiences, but also themselves when it comes to evaluating their own results."

Examine the photos carefully and scrutinize every detail, making sure that the pre- and postoperative views are identical. Look for consistency in lighting and positioning. In evaluating nasal cosmetic surgery, for example, both the before and the after side views must be identical profiles to properly judge the precise contouring change. Concentrate on the changes in facial structure that surgery has made vs. improvement in hairstyles and makeup. Compare feature with feature. Line against line. Your eyes should be going back and forth as if watching a tennis match. Be slow and deliberate. Look to see if you detect any incisions. Finally, ask yourself if you would be happy with the same degree of improvement evidenced by the people in the photos.

BEFORE SURGERY:
GETTING THE BEST FROM YOUR DOCTOR
AND HIS STAFF
Karel Rall, Patient Counselor

Our practice always schedules a preoperative visit two to three weeks prior to the procedure. Here are some of the reasons this meeting is very important.

- This is an opportunity to revisit any issues, concerns, worries and questions you may have, such as "How will my friend know what time to pick me up from the surgery center and take me home?" (Answer: At the preoperative visit, we take your friend's phone number. The surgery center's staff will call to advise of the anticipated pick-up time.) "What happens if I start to get anxious a few days before surgery?" (Answer: Dr. Kotler will prescribe a mild tranquilizer.)

- This final visit, before surgery, allows us to exchange information that we need to ensure your comfort and safety through the whole process.

- This is when we get the location and phone number of where you will be staying the night prior to surgery so that we, or your anesthesiologist, can reach you if there is a last minute change in the surgery schedule.

- This is when you should provide the name and phone numbers of the person(s) who will be staying with you after surgery.

- We will need the phone number of your pharmacy, in case special medicines need to be ordered.

● This is your chance to convey any special considerations the doctor-anesthesiologist needs to be reminded of, such as: "I get claustrophobic. Do I have assurance that Dr. Kotler calls my husband right after the surgery to tell him everything is okay." I jot down any requests you make; the reminder note goes to the front of the chart and I verbally remind Dr. Kotler about it on the evening prior to your surgery.

If you want to meet with Dr. Kotler one more time before surgery, that's perfectly fine. I'll make time in his schedule. Our office policy is: "Any question is a good question. Ask away."

I don't mind getting older; I just don't want to look it!
-Ron Sheldon, professional golfer

INSIDER'S INSIGHT
Doctor Shows Patients Before And After Photos.
You Assume They are His, But Are They?

Several months ago, a trade organization that promotes the economic interests of its members devised a program to facilitate promtional lectures/seminars by it members to the general public.

This "canned" slide presentation demonstrating facial and body cosmetic surgery is sold for $450. Accompanied by a smoothly-worded script, the 111 slides include many before and after shots of common cosmetic surgeries of the face and neck and the body. The purpose of this read-to-go program is to provide the buyer with an instant public lecture/seminar that will attract patients to that doctor's practice.

A full-page ad, promoting this package in a leading medical journal proclaims: "Each presentation is customized with your portrait photo and practice information." The ad then recommends,: "Use in your office as a continual loop in your waiting room or as a Power Point presentation for your next patient seminar!"

Can you imagine a would-be cosmetic surgeon selling his services to prospective patients, but showing another doctor's work? Is this proper? Certainly, the audience assumes it will be viewing the speaker's work, not that of another surgeon. Does the speaker disclose to the audience, up front: "These are not my cases. I bought these slides?"

Why does the speaker not have his own work to display? He should. If he does not have a portfolio of credible results, is he qualified to present himself in a public lecture as a capable cosmetic surgeon?

At a Liz Claiborne runway show, are the models dressed in Armani?

When a doctor who purports to be an accomplished cosmetic surgeon addresses the public and is directly soliciting business, the audience expects to see what he can accomplish. Examples of the art form should belong to the speaker—not to anonymous cosmetic surgeons who sell their wares through stock catalogs to doctors who do not have their own samples to present.

-RK

Whatever you may look like, marry a man your own age—as your beauty fades, so will his eyesight.

-Phyllis Diller

6

The
PHOTO GALLERY

Befores and Afters of the Most Common Procedures

THIS CHAPTER ILLUSTRATES THE MOST COMMON COSMETIC PROCEDURES in alphabetical order and provides a thumbnail description that will help you better evaluate what you are examining. Following each section are additional, procedure-specific questions you will want to ask the prospective surgeon.

BODY PROCEDURES*

AUTHOR'S NOTE: Because I perform cosmetic surgery on the face and neck only, I am not an expert on body sculpture procedures: breast surgery, liposuction, or tummy tucks. The basic information I present to you, in this chapter, was gleaned from the excellent public education brochures provided by the American Society of Plastic Surgeons. These sections were reviewed and edited for accuracy and completeness by Les Bolton, MD, FACS, a member of the Cosmetic Surgery Specialists Medical Group of Beverly Hills and Clinical Instructor of Plastic Surgery, USC School of Medicine.

BREAST AUGMENTATION
(Augmentation Mammaplasty)

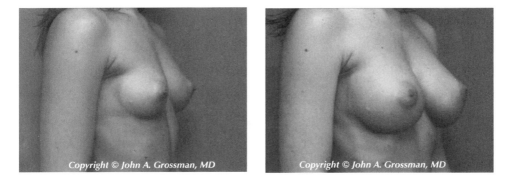

Breast Augmentation
Photos courtesy of John A. Grossman, MD.

This procedure enhances the size and improves the shape of a woman's breast. It may enhance the body contour of a woman whose breast size is inadequate, create a balance between different breast sizes, correct a reduced breast volume after pregnancy, or reconstruct a breast following cancer surgery.

> **More women than ever before had breast augmentation surgery in 2000. Breast augmentation increased 476 percent since 1992, 42 percent since 1999.**
>
> **-The 2001 Report of the 2000 Procedural Statistics, American Society of Plastic Surgeons***

There are several kinds of breast implants. All implants have a silicone plastic shell, but are filled with either liquid silicone gel or a special saline (salt water) solution. Some implants have been modified to have a "balloon within a balloon" permitting some adjustments in size during surgery. Other implants have a textured surface presumably to encourage stronger bonding between the surrounding natural tissue and the implant, reducing the chance of an internal scarring. Your doctor should be conversant in the pros and cons of various implants for your specific needs.

*ASPS Procedural Statistics represent procedures performed by ASPS member plastic surgeons certified by the American Board of Plastic Surgery, as well as other physicians certified by the American Board of Medical Specialties-recognized boards.

There are several routes of insertion. The most direct way is through a curved incision in the crease between the breast and the chest, though many surgeons prefer to insert through a hidden incision, either around the nipple or through the armpit. Techniques have recently been developed for insertion of breast implants through a distant incision at the navel, although longevity and positioning may be problematic. Further, the implants may be placed at different levels Some surgeons place the implant directly under the breast tissue, others beneath the chest wall muscle. The route of insertion and location of the incisions are not as important as how symmetrical and centered the breasts are after the procedure.

Typically, the operation is performed as an outpatient procedure under general anesthesia. Surface stitches, if used, are removed within seven to ten days. Compression dressings may be used for several days and minor soreness is controlled with pain medication. Body incisions tend to take a bit longer to heal than incisions of the face and neck. Scars may be firm and pink for six weeks. After several months they fade and become rather inconspicuous.

Questions to Ask if You Are Considering Breast Augmentation:

- Silicone-filled implants look and feel very natural. They were once thought to be associated with unusual autoimmune diseases until scientific studies proved otherwise. Can I have them if I want them?

- If my breasts are not symmetrical after surgery, what can be done?

- I have seen some implants that look very unnatural—they look like they are right under the skin. Is this condition a function of the type of implant, or its placement?

- If I do not want any visible scars, what is my best option?

- Is it dangerous to put implants under the chest muscle near the rib cage?

- I heal poorly with thick scars. Is there a greater risk of capsule thickening for me?

- As I get older, will my breasts sag more with implants? If so, what can be done?

- If I gain weight and my breasts enlarge, will they become saggy?

- Will implants make it harder for my doctor to detect breast cancer? Do implants compromise the value of mammograms?

- What happens if an implant ruptures or leaks? How will I know? How will my breasts look? What can be done?

- If I get an infection, does the breast implant have to come out? What about the other implant? If it stays, will I look funny?

- After surgery, how long before I can engage in strenuous exercise? How long before I can have sex?

- What if I am not happy with the size of my implants? Can they be "exchanged"?

- What is the most common complication of breast enlargement? How is this handled?

- What is the most serious complication?

- Some Hollywood people have obvious "boob jobs" and look grotesque. Do they look this way because of their own poor judgment, the surgeon's judgment or a combination of both?

At the beginning of my shift, I placed a stethoscope on an elderly and slightly deaf female patient's anterior chest wall. "Big breaths," I instructed.

"Yes, they used to be," the patient said sadly.

-Doctors Have Good Sories Too,
from Dr. S. Schrader, via Dr. H.A.W. Kriger

BREAST REDUCTION
(Reduction Mammaplasty)

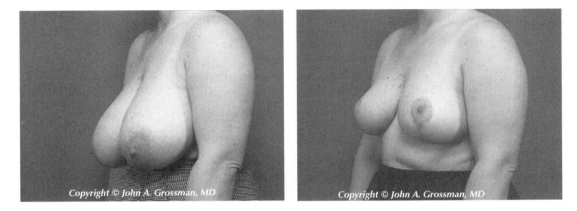

Copyright © John A. Grossman, MD   *Copyright © John A. Grossman, MD*

Breast Reduction
Photos courtesy of John A. Grossman, MD.

Women with excessively large breasts suffer a variety of problems—both physical and psychological. A breast reduction may be indicated if the patient experiences chronic neck and back pain, skin irritations or indentations from bra straps. The psychological burden accompanying unusually large breasts can be just as harmful, particularly in younger women who may have difficulty finding clothing or participating in physical activities others take for granted.

Breast reduction surgery removes fat, glandular breast tissue, and skin as a unit, making the breasts smaller, lighter and firmer. The nipple and areola are also lifted as a part of the procedure. The objective is to achieve better proportion between a woman's breasts and her body.

Because heavy breasts can lead to medical problems including skeletal deformities and breathing problems, many women request breast reduction surgery. Breast reduction surgery relieves pain in the back, neck and shoulders. Beyond the medical problems it allows women to feel more comfortable in clothing and more importantly— with themselves. Last year, breast reduction surgery was performed on 84,780 women.

-The 2001 Report of the 2000 Procedural Statistics,
American Society of Plastic Surgeons

This procedure is more extensive than breast augmentation. Although the location of the operation is dependent upon your doctor's evaluation, it will likely be done in a hospital where the proper equipment and blood for potential transfusion is accessible. Breast reduction is usually performed under general anesthesia, but you will usually return home the same day.

While there are a variety of techniques, the traditional procedure usually involves an anchor-shaped incision that circles the nipple, extends downward, and then follows both to the left and right of the natural crease beneath the breast. It does leave permanent scars, although they are placed to be as inconspicuous as possible. After removing skin and underlying breast tissue, the remaining tissue is brought together and the wound is closed with multiple layers of stitches. In most cases, the nipples remain attached to the blood vessels and nerves so sensation is unaffected. (There are rare situations where the nipples have to be completely removed and grafted to a higher location.)

Suction tubes stay in place for one or two days to remove blood and fluid. This reduces swelling and bruising, hastening recovery. Often a special elastic bandage or custom surgical bra is used to apply gentle pressure to the healing tissue.

The patient can expect to resume normal activity within two weeks. Those wanting to engage in strenuous exercise—particularly involving the upper body—must refrain for an additional one to two weeks. Scars may take up to six months before maturing and becoming less obvious.

Questions to Ask if You Are Considering Breast Reduction:

- Will breast reduction influence my ability to breast-feed?

- Can anything be done if I am disappointed in my breasts' shape or size after surgery?

- What if my nipples are not at the same level, or point differently after surgery? Can this be fixed?

- If I develop thick unsightly scars, how can they be improved?

- What are my options if my nipple must be grafted and could potentially die? What can be done?

- My friend had to get a mammogram before breast reduction surgery. Why?

- I was advised to get "liposuction of the armpit" at the same time as my breast reduction. Can you explain why?

- What are the chances I will need a blood transfusion? Can you donate my own blood ahead of time?

- What are the factors indicating hospital surgery?

- My heavy breasts cause chronic neck and back pain. Will insurance pay for my surgery?

- How long must I wait for the swelling to go down so I can see the final result?

BREAST LIFT
(Mastopexy)

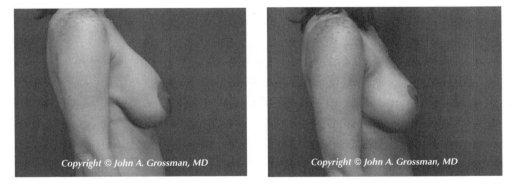

Breast Lift without implants
Photos courtesy of John A. Grossman, MD.

This procedure is designed to literally lift sagging breasts without major removal of tissue or the insertion of implants. Sagging breasts are often the result of multiple pregnancies during which time the breasts enlarged but could not contract to the original pre-pregnancy state. This procedure involves removal of some portion of skin to allow the breast tissue to be repositioned higher. Technical details are similar to that for breast reduction discussed above. Some circumstances dictate that breast implants may enhance overall appearance. This should be addressed during your consultation.

LIPOSUCTION
(Lipoplasty)

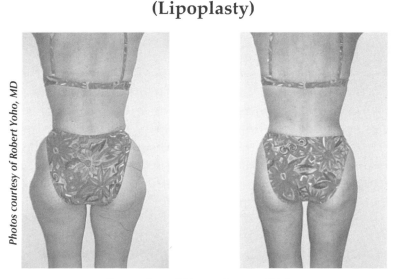

Photos courtesy of Robert Yoho, MD

Liposuction of hips and upper thighs

Liposuction is the most popular plastic surgery among women, according to the American Society of Plastic Surgeons. It is also called suction-assisted lipectomy, suction lipectomy or fat suction. This procedure, devised by a French gynecologist in response to a patient's prodding, used the suction apparatus reserved for rapid abortions to "get rid of fat."

> **Liposuction procedures increased 386 percent between 1992 and 2000.**
>
> *-The 2001 Report of the 2000 Procedural Statistics* **American Society of Plastic Surgeons**

The technique removed unwanted fat deposits from specific areas of the body including upper arms, chest, abdomen, buttocks, hips, thighs, knees, calves and ankles. *Liposuction is not a substitute for legitimate weight reduction programs,* but rather a method of removing localized fat that won't respond to dieting and exercise. Since the newly formed contour is dependent upon contraction of the overlying skin, the best candidates for liposuction are those patients who are young with good skin quality and not obese.

Liposuction is almost always an outpatient procedure. The location can be a properly outfitted office, outpatient surgery center or hospital. It can be done under local anesthesia, local anesthesia with sedation or general anesthesia. Very small incisions are made to insert the vacuum-suction tube underneath the skin. These are deliberately placed in inconspicuous locations. Following surgery, a snug girdle or body stocking is worn over the treated areas to reduce swelling and bruising and encourage your skin to conform to the new underlying architecture. The garment may have to be worn for several weeks. Though return to work and normal duties takes place within a few days, strenuous exercise may be uncomfortable for two to four weeks following the procedure.

> **Liposuction was the most popular cosmetic surgical procedure among women with 302,236 performed.**
>
> *-The 2001 Report of the 2000 Procedural Statistics,* **American Society of Plastic Surgeons**

A variety of modifications regarding technique and equipment design have been adopted since liposuction was first introduced in the United States in the 1980s. These refinements have made the procedure less traumatic and produce better results. Over time, much smaller suction tubes evolved minimizing incisions and improving the evenness of the suctioning. Several years ago, researchers developed Ultrasound-Assisted Lipoplasty (UAL) whereby fat is liquefied prior to suction removal for better contouring. Power-Assisted Lipoplasty (PAL) has recently been introduced where fat is more easily removed through vibration of the suction tube. This procedure however, has the potential to cause lumpiness, particularly in the hands of less experienced surgeons. The most recent modification is known as Vaser-Assisted Lipoplasty (VAL) where intermittent sound waves liquefy the fat, allowing for a more rapid and precise process. All of these recent advances are advantageous for some, but not all, patient situations.

Questions To Ask If You Are Considering Liposuction:

- Is there an age limit for liposuction?

- Are certain areas of the body where skin elasticity is poor less satisfactory for liposuction?

- If major liposuction is performed, will I need a blood transfusion? Should I "bank" my own blood?

- Should large volume liposuction be done in the hospital?

- My skin forms keloid scars. How big an issue is this for liposuction?

● Should I expect dimpling of the skin after liposuction?

● If one gains weight after liposuction, what happens to the previously liposuctioned areas? Will the areas that have not been treated tend to show greater evidence of weight gain? Will I look strange?

● Can an area be liposuctioned more than once?

TUMMY TUCK
(Abdominoplasty)

Tummy Tuck
Photos courtesy of John A. Grossman, MD.

This procedure classified as major cosmetic surgery, removes excess skin and fat from the mid and lower abdomen. Abdominal muscles may also be tightened as part of the procedure. The objective of this surgery is to correct a protruding abdomen caused by pregnancy or genetic predisposition. The degree of surgery is dependent upon the amount of excess tissue in place; therefore patients who intend to lose (a significant amount of) weight should postpone surgery. Likewise, women planning future pregnancies may want to defer the procedure particularly when seeking to tighten their abdominals. These could separate during the "stretching" process of pregnancy. The appearance of existing abdominal scars may worsen.

Surgeons perform this operation in a hospital or a properly equipped and accredited outpatient surgery center. It is always done under general anesthesia. The operation may take two to five hours.

Tummy tuck procedures increased 227 percent since 1992.

-The 2001 Report of the 2000 Procedural Statistics, **American Society of Plastic Surgeons**

Because of the major tissue movement, healing time and wound quality may vary in individuals. Cigarette smoking and/or poor circulation will have an adverse effect and hence add greater risk.

The long incision is closed in layers using both deep (hidden) stitches and either surface stitches or surgical clips. A suction drain-tube is usually inserted for two to five days to reduce swelling and bruising and aid in healing.

A special support and compression garment is usually worn for a week or so. While most patients can return to work and resume normal activities in two weeks, it may take a bit longer for some. Exercise programs can be safely resumed in three to four weeks. Scar maturation can take up to nine months, which is typical for any operation done on the abdomen.

Questions to Ask if You Are Considering a Tummy Tuck:

- What factors determine if correction of my abdominal fullness can be accomplished by liposuction vs. a tummy tuck?

- What is a "partial" or "mini tummy tuck"? Am I a candidate?

- What happens if I gain weight after? Lose weight?

- Can problems occur if I become pregnant after surgery?

- What are the chances of keloid scars?

- I do a strenuous workout program including sit-ups. How long before I can resume these activities?

- What is the most common complication? How is it corrected?

- What is the most serious complication? How is this handled?

Face and Neck Procedures*

CHEEK IMPLANTS
(Malarplasty)

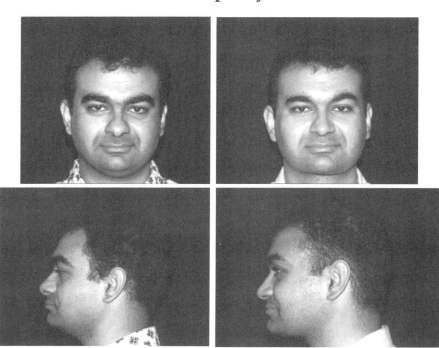

Cheek implants, neck sculpture plus nasal cosmetic surgery
Les Bolton, MD, FACS, performed the cheek augmentation.

Some men and women, to improve and achieve facial structure, benefit from "cheek implants." Cheek implantation is analogous to chin implantation. Solid, silicone, plastic, FDA-approved, preformed "parts" are placed onto the existing cheekbones, beneath the surface, to give more satisfactory prominence to the cheek areas. There are two routes of insertion: through a linear incision fashioned under the lower eyelid lashes (often used for lower eyelid and/or other midfacial surgeries, also), or through hidden incisions in the mouth, placed above the gum line on the face of the upper jaw bone, hidden by the upper lip.

*All photos in this section are courtesy of Dr. Kotler's office.

The challenge for the surgeon is to create normal appearing cheek prominences that are approximately symmetrical. "One high and one low" is a no-no because it will be obvious and unsatisfactory. And, as with chin augmentation, underdoing is better than overdoing.

Make sure the doctor who proposes this procedure is experienced and can show many technically-identical "before and after" photo examples.

Questions You Need to Ask if You Are Considering Cheek Implantation:

- May I see the implant you suggest?

- Why do you recommend this particular style, shape and size for me?

- What is the chance of "slippage" or rejection? Will this cause damage to my tissues?

- What route of insertion do you recommend? Why?

- If the cheek implants are inserted through the mouth, is there a greater chance of infection?

- If inserted via a lower eyelid incision, can the eyelids be injured or malformed by the implant surgery?

- How are implants anchored or kept in place?

- Will there by numbness of the face and/or lips? If so, for how long?

- If one or both of the implants ever have to be removed, when can they be replaced?

CHIN AUGMENTATION
(Mentoplasty)

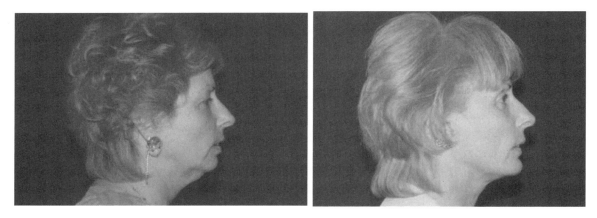

Upper eyelids and chin augmentation combined with neck sculpture give maximum profile improvement.

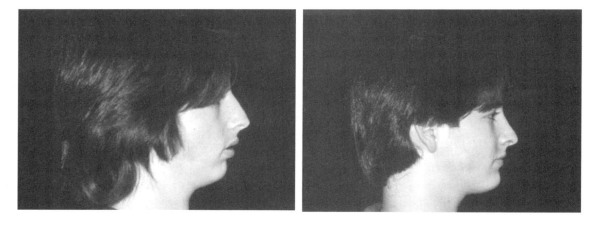

This young man had correction of receding chin and nasal surgery.

Correction of a receding chin is frequently performed simultaneously with face and neck lifting, neck sculpturing or nasal cosmetic surgery. Today's techniques utilize plastic inserts that are quite safe and not likely to dislodge. They may be inserted through the mouth or through a fine incision hidden under the chin (discussed later in Face and Neck lifting). The latter technique is preferred by most surgeons.

The key word describing the successful chin augmentation is "natural." Too large an implant will look unnatural; too small an insert will leave the patient with little difference in appearance. Implants should be centered and secured at the time of placement to avoid an asymmetrical appearance.

Questions You Need to Ask if You Are Considering Chin Augmentation:

- What kind of implant material is used to build up the chin? Is it safe? Is it FDA approved? Can I see one?

- How long have these implants been used?

- How are they inserted?

- What is the chance of "rejection"? If the implant is being rejected, how is it managed? Will this cause damage to my tissues?

- What are the chances of infection? What if this happens to me?

- Is there a possibility the implant can shift position? If this happened, what do we do? If the implant has to be removed for any reason, can it be replaced later? How long an interval must I wait?

CORRECTION OF PROTRUDING EARS
(Otoplasty)

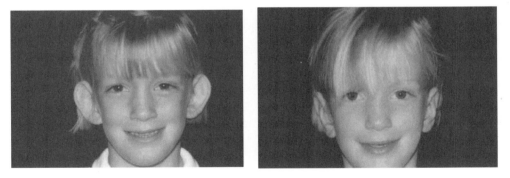

These photos tell the story.

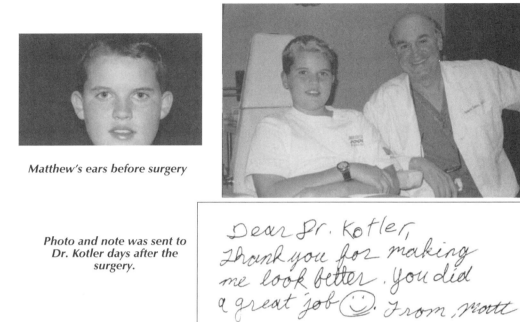

Matthew's ears before surgery

Photo and note was sent to Dr. Kotler days after the surgery.

Dear Dr. Kotler,
Thank you for making
me look better. You did
a great job ☺. From, Matt

Ear position can be corrected on adults or on children five years or older. The objective of the surgery is to permanently recontour the pliable ear cartilage. This is done by sculpting and reshaping the cartilage through incisions hidden on the back surface of the ear.

Well-performed surgery will yield natural appearing ears. The visible contours should be smooth and gentle without any sharp edges. A "pulled" or "pinned-back" look is not necessary. No incisions should be visible and both ears should be nearly identical. Expect a 3-5 day recovery.

Questions You Need to Ask if You Are Considering Ear Correction:

- Is there a difference between the child's and the adult's operation?

- What will keep my ears closer to my head? Will they "pull out" after a period of time?

- One ear is different from the other. Can they be made exactly the same?

- How bad is the swelling? When do you think I can appear in public without any dressing?

- Does the operation have any effect upon my hearing?

- I have big earlobes. Can they be made smaller?

- I understand the ears are "numb" for a time after surgery. Can you explain why and how long this numbness will last?

EYELID SURGERY
(Blepharoplasty)

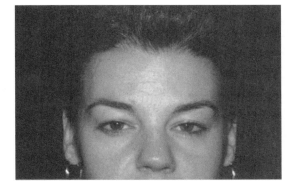 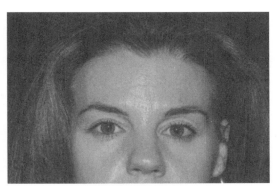

Upper and lower eyelid surgery
See Mishel's letter in Chapter 11 — page 223.

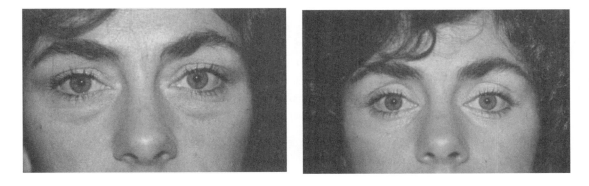

Eyelid surgery lightens and brightens.

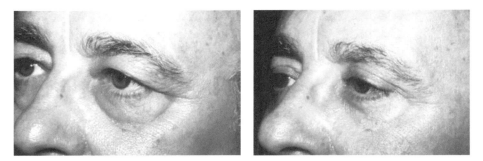

Male eyelid surgery — the secret of success is not overdoing.

The objective of upper eyelid surgery is to remove the fold of the skin that forms between the eyelash and eyebrow, which conceals the natural eyelid and obscures the cleft that separates the lid from the brow. Eyes appear "hooded." This profound pleat-like fold of skin may interfere with normal vision when it becomes heavy.

PATIENT COMMENTARY

This letter is to express my satisfaction with my recent eye surgery and report back to you the results in terms of the change in my life after making a decision to have this procedure. The procedure itself went very smoothly and I could see clearly enough to get around in only a few days. Within three to four weeks, I looked like a more awake and vigorous version of my old self. The change is exactly what I want in that I still look like my old self, only better, more alert and younger. The general opinion of my friends was that I look different but they could not quite decide what was different, except I look more awake and younger. I redoubled my career search, with extra confidence and I'm happy to report that I now have the highest and best paying computer sales position in my industry…Appearance in how you both feel and present yourself is a part of life and taking action to improve yourself simply makes good sense.

-Brandt, sales executive, Tennessee

Standard upper lid surgery removes this excess skin and fatty tissue through an incision neatly placed in that natural crease between the eyelid and eyebrow. The incision can be fashioned using a specific

As the nation ages, surgeries such as eyelid cosmetic surgery have grown common—increasing by 139% between 1992 and 1999. Forehead and brow lifts...increasing by 203% during the same time period.

-USC Health,
Spring 2001

laser beam or a conventional scalpel technique. The end result is the same in either case. These incisions should become nearly (or completely) invisible within a short period of time. Even though the lids are somewhat "tight" at first, they gradually relax and assume normal function. Symmetry between right and left sides is extremely important to the success of the operation.

Lower eyelid surgery is performed primarily to remove "bags" caused by bulging fatty tissue beneath the skin. One incision for removal of fatty tissue and/or skin is made very close to the lower lashes and extends into one of the crow's feet or laugh lines. These incisions heal rapidly and are barely visible. An option for some younger patients is to remove only fatty tissue through an internal incision behind the lower lid. The surgeon's choice of incision depends on various factors determined by examination. Upper and lower eyelid cosmetic surgery can be performed independently of one another or together.

Questions To Ask If You Are Considering Upper Eyelid Surgery:

- Does the eyebrow have to be lifted with every upper eyelid surgery?

- I've heard that some people have trouble closing their eyes after upper eyelid surgery. Why does this happen? How is it corrected? Will this happen to me?

- My upper eyelids are so heavy that my vision is impaired. This being the case, does my operation qualify for insurance benefits? What steps must we take to have my insurance company approve the procedure?

- What are the advantages and disadvantages of laser vs. traditional surgery?

- How soon can I wear my contact lenses after eyelid surgery?

Questions to Ask if You Are Considering Lower Eyelid Surgery:

- I have extra skin and "puffiness" under my eyes. How are each of these problems managed?

- If I have wrinkled skin, how is that usually treated?

- What is "laser eyelid surgery"? How does it differ from traditional surgery? What are the advantages and disadvantages?

- Based upon my appearance, am I a candidate for the external or internal incisions?

FACE AND NECK LIFTING
(Cervicofacial Rhytidectomy)

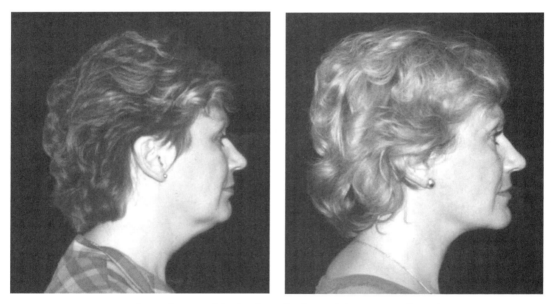

Note the sculpture of the jowls and substantial, yet natural result.

Face and neck lifting offer several alternatives because you are dealing with multiple components. Common procedures include tightening under the chin or about the neck, sculpting the jawline and cheeks, or removal of jowls. While individual procedures may vary somewhat, certain standards apply in all cases. Certain features of face and neck lifting are visible to the trained eye. The following includes information on incisions, and tips on evaluation of the work on the neck and jawline:

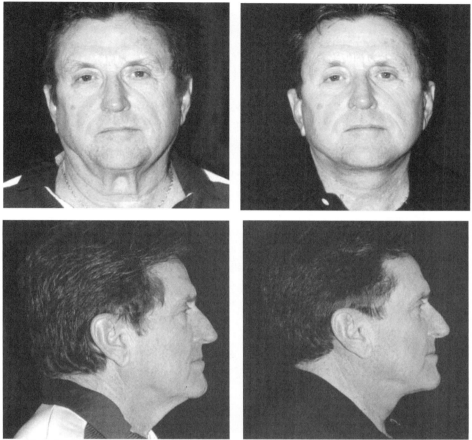

Male face and neck lift...the emphasis is on tighting the sagging neck and restoring a sharp jaw line. Conservatively done—not pulled. This gentleman saw how great his wife looked (she is on page 135) and decided he could improve as well!

Face-lift techniques of the past often left vertical, wide incision-scars with "railroad tie" cross-hatchings. These were poorly placed in front of the ear, onto the cheek, and were visible unless camouflaged by hairstyle. Contemporary surgeons now fashion two incisions in two different locations. The first, a single, curving incision above the ear, permits access so that the forehead, brow, cheeks, jawline and neck can be tightened.

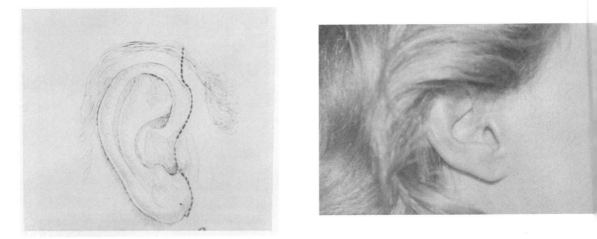

It is critical that the visible portion of the incision be concealed. The curved incision is camouflaged by the folds of the external ear. The remaining invisible portions of the incision are hidden behind the ear.

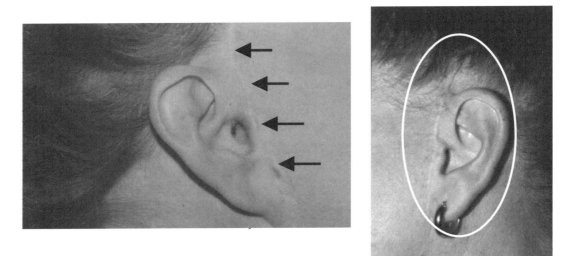

Conspicuous, poorly placed incisions — right ear & left ear

Location and pattern of incisions differ somewhat by gender. For females, it begins within the hairline of the temple, then continues downward within the various creases and curves of the ear. That nasty, straight-line, vertical, white and widened scar—visible well in front of the ear—mentioned earlier, is avoided using this pattern. The incision continues behind the earlobe, into the groove behind the ear, and then terminates horizontally within the hairline.

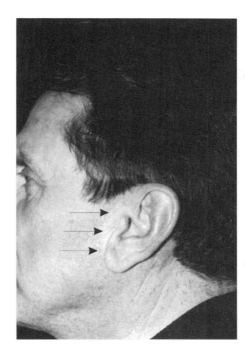

Male incision hugs the back edge of the sideburn and continues just behind the earlobe.

PATIENT COMMENTARY

After my face and neck lift, I can now button my collar, without my face falling over the collar. Before, I had to gather up my neck.

- Michael, actor, California

The male incision also begins within the temple hairline, hugs the back edge of the sideburn and then continues downward to just below the earlobe. It is important that the incision's slightly bowed, vertical portion in front of the ear, be precisely placed at the junction of the back edge of the sideburn, and the hairless strip of skin, just in front of the ear. This natural boundary is the best location to camouflage the incision. Were the male incisions identical to that of the female—hidden in the folds and contours of the ear—shaving would be a challenge. Further, with the beard growing at the ear canal opening, an unnatural appearance will be unforgivingly permanent. The male's incision—hidden behind the ear and in the hairline—is identical to the female's.

More experienced surgeons generally required less time to perform a face lift.

-National Plastic Surgery Survey journal *Plastic and Reconstructive Surgery*, October 2000

Patients who heal satisfactorily can expect their incisions to be completely hidden or obscured. The fully healed wound should become a fine, nearly imperceptible line, particularly in that portion that hugs the ear. In patients with very thin, fair skin, the incision may be completely invisible. Today, because of better-placed incisions, women can wear their hair "up," baring their ears without fear of revealing telltale incisions. Even for men, with fewer hairstyle options, incisions are well concealed and acceptable.

The second incision is used to remove the double chin and correct the hanging, vertical platysma muscle bands in the neck (the so-called "turkey neck"). This horizontal, fine-line incision is well hidden—where chin meets neck—and is almost always, ultimately, invisible. As desired, a chin implant (see Chin Augmentation) can be placed through this incision, to further accentuate the new jawline.

The objective of face and neck lifting is to restore a youthful appearance to the face and neck. From the front, erasing the jowls and removing the hanging, often floppy vertical muscle bands reverses those telltale signs of aging evidenced in the mirror.

There Are Three Common Techniques for Neck and Face lifting

There are three main variations of the face and neck lift:

- skin or subcutaneous lift
- the SMAS lift
- the deep plane lift.

Each is defined by the layers of facial tissue and muscles that are shifted to attain "the lift."

The skin or subcutaneous (under the skin) lift focuses on removing excess skin and redraping the remaining skin while sculpting the excess fatty tissue of the jowls and neck below the jaw line. This is the venerable and most traditional of the procedures.

The SMAS lift focuses on the anatomically defined layer of covering tissue below the fat and intimately related to the muscle covering. The aim is to "lift" the deeper layers, beneath the skin and fatty tissue. This technique was first performed in the late 1970s after anatomists discovered the significance of this layer of tissue—called the SMAS—and its implications for face-lifting. The hope invested in this procedure was that it would have greater longevity; however, a solidly researched recent journal article concluded that this variation added no greater lifespan value to the classical skin/ subcutaneous lift.

A decade later, the **deep plane lift** techniques evolved. Attempting to release the lift burden from the skin, and hoping for the longer lasting result, surgeons began burrowing deep under the skin, fat, SMAS, and facial muscles of expression. Lifting these, as a unit, would hopefully reduce the chances of skin overstretching with its negative consequences and yet give a more durable result. Some consider this the most radical of the face-lifting options because of the risk of the overtightened, overlifted, "always surprised" appearance, usually due to the overly aggressive repositioning of eyes and brows.

Each procedure and its minor modifications have advantages and disadvantages. Each has its own set of potential complications, problems and dissatisfactions. Be sure to ask each surgeon you interview to recommend the technique appropriate for you—*in his hands—and why.* Then, make sure you understand what will be done. And, do not leave that office until you see many *before* and *after* photos of patients whose *befores* illustrate the same types of dissatisfactions that you want solved.

Finally, please remember that face lifts—of any variety—cannot transform wrinkled, lined, weather-beaten, aged-spotted skin to youthful, smooth, fresh skin. Only resurfacing—chemical or laser—does that. Surgery to "pull out" wrinkles never works. It can even nullify the success of an appropriate lift. And, when you see that unfortunate man or woman whose face is in a perpetual smile, or suggests they just ended a ride strapped to the tail of a 747, you will know they were never told that surgery is always the wrong solution for wrinkles. And you will know they never had the opportunity and the wisdom to read this book.

What the mirror cannot demonstrate is your profile: that poor definition between jaw and neck, the sagging and blending together. A high quality face and necklift restores the lost angulation between the jawline and the neck by evacuation of the fatty jowls, and trimming and tightening the lax, vertical platysma neck muscle.

These procedures form an internal corset. Repositioning those vertical bands, in the front of the neck, will recreate a more satisfactory angle between the chin and neck. The redundant skin is redraped and the excess is removed, not from the "front" but from the "back," through the hidden incision behind the ear and in the hairline. Removing major amounts of excess skin from the front of the face or neck is out of

---

 **INSIDER'S INSIGHT**

A Face Lift Every Three To Four Years? Get Real

I am astonished when some well-heeled, Beverly Hills matron proudly announces she has had multiple face lifts. My guess is she has confused quantity with quality. It is no badge of honor to have the major facial cosmetic surgery that often. There is no value there either. We expect our face and neck lifts to last ten to fifteen years or longer. Just recently, we did a "second lift" for one of our patients whose first was 21 years earlier. She is not unhappy about having the second lift; she had a good run with the first. And after surgery, she kiddingly said, "Well, if I get 21 years out of this one, I'll be back when I'm 81 years of age. I'll probably still be around because my mother's in her 90's. Dr. Kotler, will you be here?"

I sure hope so, Mary Anne.

-RK

> **Face-lifts for aging have to be subtle . . . you can't have total rejuvenation and still keep the integrity of the face.**
>
> **- Joan Kron, author**
> *Lift: Wanting, Fearing, and Having a Face-lift*

the question because it would require a long, visible incision.

Surgical face and neck lifting should not be employed to remove wrinkles or age spots. These imperfections are corrected via a chemical or laser process described later. Surgically pulling or stretching wrinkled facial skin will be no more successful than attempting to "iron" a wrinkled shirt by stretching the fabric.

Poorly performed surgery of face and neck can announce itself in one of two ways. The first will be a consequence of undertreatment of jowls: a double chin, vertical neck folds, or sagging cheeks, brows and temples. Complaints from patients might be that "my face and neck dropped again, only several months after surgery." Usually, this is a result of the original surgery doing little more than tightening the skin, the so-called "minilift." Incidentally my motto is "minilift equals miniresult." More aggressive, modern techniques correct the beneath-the-skin muscle sag and fat accumulation yielding better results that last far longer.

The second possible advertisement of a poorly performed face and neck lift will be that overly tight distortion of facial features. The artificial look. Patients will complain of a "plastic" or "drum-like" appearance. Too much was done; the opposite of the minilift. This unfortunate appearance is the consequence of inappropriate, over-zealous, mis-directed face tightening. Usually, an unrealistic, vain attempt to erase wrinkles and lines about the cheeks, mouth and eyes. The "nasolabial fold," between the cheeks and the upper lip and nose, is very difficult to eradicate even by the most aggressive techniques. While drastic tightening temporarily smoothes out these wrinkles lines and grooves, the effect is short-lived. The skin is elastic, like a rubber band, and will contract, causing all such dissatisfactions to return. Further, vigorous tightening is risky since the incisions can break down or later can heal with thick unattractive scars.

Face Lifts and Weight Loss

If you are a bit overweight, should you lose weight? I say yes, but before—not after—the trip to the operating room. I prefer to see the patient at their ideal weight for two important reasons:

INSIDER'S INSIGHT

We always give our patients our best efforts, but sometimes to get the best result, we need YOUR help. Waiting six months for surgery while you sustain a healthful weight loss is a reasonable price for a safer better, longer-lasting result.

-RK

- Obesity is a health risk and complicates the anesthetic. The anesthesiologist's job is tough enough without the stress of attending to someone who is overweight.

- While we can successfully sculpt excess superficial fat from beneath the skin of the jaw and neckline, we have no access to deeper layers of fatty tissue. Weight loss will shrink that deep fat and increase the success of the facelift.

I advise patients to pursue a slow, constant weight-loss program, ideally under medical supervision, and then return in six months for a reevaluation.

As you probably guessed, weight loss after surgery makes no sense. The good tightening achieved can be seriously compromised because the fatty tissue under the freshly redraped and tightened skin will shrink. The skin then relaxes and the benefits of the surgery are lost.

Patients' greatest fear is this windblown, over-tightened, strange, unnatural facelift. It does not have to be that way. Such an appearance is never the result of patient request; rather, it is the hallmark of an amateur cosmetic surgeon. It does not satisfy the patient's wish to look better, rather than different. Scan the doctor's album closely; look for improvement that looks proper and natural, not strange, artificial or abnormal. When you see lots of results that would satisfy you, you're viewing work by a serious cosmetic surgeon with good judgment.

Allison Hatfield states in her *Fort Worth* article "He's So Vain," that a face lift is trickier for men than for women. "In general, male facial skin has a richer blood supply than female facial skin. Men bleed more during facial surgery and have a greater chance of hematoma, a temporary pooling of blood under the skin during or after surgery. Scarring may be more difficult for men to hide, as most do not wear make-up or style their hair towards their faces as women do. Men with thinning hair may require a bit more surgical artistry to hide scars, especially in the temple area. When a guy has a face lift, his hair and beard may play a role in its outcome. Hair-bearing skin of the upper neck may be pulled behind the ears, meaning some guys will end up having to shave behind their ears or suffer through electrolysis."

> *"His face is pulled so tight, that when he smiles, his arms go up"!*
> -Hal Jay, WBAP radio, Dallas, Texas,
> describing a prominent Dallas citizen's recent
> (overdone) cosmetic surgery

Specific Questions to Ask if You Are Considering a Face and Neck Lift:

- Do you do that "deep plane" facelift? Is it appropriate for me? If you do not do "deep plane," how do you lift the sagging facial tissue? Will skin be removed?

- How will the neck be managed? Is there a separate neck incision? Where? Does the sagging platysma muscle need attention?

- Do you place suction drains? If so, why? For how long? Where do they exit? How are they removed? Is it painful?

- How long do you expect the face-lift procedure to "last"? What factors might cause less longevity? Is the second procedure as extensive? How might it be different?

- I've seen people who look like they "walked behind a jet engine." The face had a "pulled" look. What is the reason for that? Can you assure me that I will not have a similar result?

- Does every facelift include eyelid surgery and/or forehead and eyebrow lifting? Does every facelift include the neck?

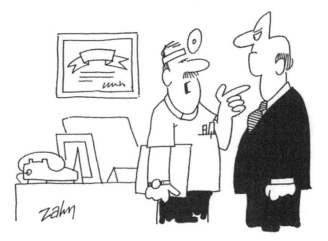

"Remember, Mr. Benton—I warned you that there's an element of risk in all face lifts."

- Why do some mature people have a "nose job" with their facelift? Is this done routinely? Is it right for me?

- I've heard that some people have a chin implant placed at the time of facelifting. Would I need to have one?

- I'm 77 years old and healthy. Am I too old for a full facelift?

- Will I lose my facial expression?

- Does a facelift correct laugh lines around the mouth, or frown lines in the forehead and between the eyes? Will it remove the groove that runs between my nose and the outer corner of my mouth?

● Will my hair be shaved off? When can I wash my hair? When can I color my hair?

FACIAL REJUVENATION
(Chemical or Laser)

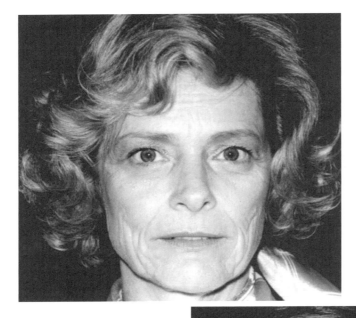

*Chemical skin peel only—
NO surgery*

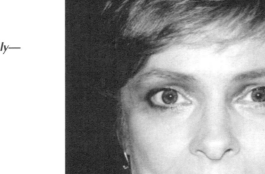

Laser And Chemical Skin Peels
Personal Experience And Observation

Having been involved with both medical lasers and chemical skin peels for nearly 30 years, I can give you a qualified opinion. My initial training in chemical peeling began in 1969 under Dr. Richard Ariagno at Northwestern University Medical School. In 1971, while at the University of Illinois College of Medicine, our department received one of the nation's first generation medical lasers. At that time we used it primarily for tumor surgery. In the early 1990s, I employed lasers in nasal surgery and major facelifting. When laser technology was adapted for use in skin resurfacing/wrinkle removal, I joined my colleagues in evaluating that "latest technique."

Lasers have intriguing potential for many uses, but questions remain, particularly concerning skin resurfacing. Do lasers measure up to the 40-year gold standard for wrinkle removal — the phenol deep chemical skin peel? And which lasers are best?

In 1991, I wrote the medical text **Chemical Rejuvenation of the Face.** Purchased primarily by cosmetic surgeons and dermatologists wanting to learn the process or improve their skills, this single-procedure textbook was well received and a medical best seller. I was quite proud when prominent dermatologic surgeon, James Fulton, MD, PhD, one of the co-formulators of Retin-A®, publicly pronounced the textbook "The Bible of Chemical Skin Peeling." In preparation, I reviewed nearly every book and medical journal article written on the subject. My research further enhanced my understanding of how skin ages and what we doctors can and cannot do about reversing that aging.

In 1998, Lawrence Moy, MD (a fellow UCLA faculty member in the Dermatology Division), and I conducted joint research comparing the newer laser technology with traditional chemical skin peeling. An independent pathologist examined both techniques side by side using microscopic skin samples from volunteer patients. This landmark study was published in a major medical journal.* It presents very strong evidence of the relative virtues and expectations for each of these treatment techniques.

-RK

So, which is "better" — laser or chemical? The answer on the surface is: "It depends." A young person in his or her 30s or early 40s, with early signs of skin aging, will probably be satisfied with a less powerful laser or mild chemical peeling agent. A 60-year-old with "crocodile skin" would require a more aggressive technique, such as deep phenol peel or high-intensity laser.

Here are some important caveats to remember. The more intensive the skin resurfacing by either process the greater the potential for prolonged healing, color

> **Wrinkles are the worst thing to get rid of – practically impossible. You _cannot_ get rid of them even with a facelift. It's a peel or nothing.**
>
> **-Joan Rivers**

---

* *Dermatologic Surgery*, November 1999.

irregularities, and even complications such as scarring. Skin tone, thickness, dryness or oiliness, depth and location of wrinkles and prior treatments are all factors that must be considered when choosing the type and strength of resurfacing. The "best" procedure is the one tailored to the individual by a highly specialized doctor who understands both the benefits and risks of laser and chemical treatments.

> **Surgical techniques of facial rejuvenation have become quite sophisticated in the past several years.... and among the many methods and techniques now offered are alpha hydroxy acids, tretinoin (Retin-A), dermabrasion, phenol peel, trichloroacetic acid peel, and resurfacing with CO2 and Erbium lasers. Facial skin has undergone a multiplicity of changes and continues to improve.**
>
> **New techniques and procedures continue to evolve rapidly and there is no doubt that what is presented in this issue will be improved upon, changed, or even discarded. The specialty of aesthetic surgery and specifically facial skin resurfacing is not static, but forever advancing. We continue to strive for perfection.**
>
> **-Thomas J. Baker, MD, FACS**
> **Guest Editor, *Clinics in Plastic Surgery, Skin Resurfacing,***
> **January 1998**

The aim of both processes is to destroy the outermost skin layers and thereby induce nature to replace the older, wrinkled, sun-damaged skin with new, smooth, unwrinkled skin, free of age spots and other precancerous areas that are the hallmark of aged skin. The ability of man to create "new skin from old skin" has been a desire since antiquity. Records show, for example, that ancient Egyptian women rubbed their facial skin with alabaster stone in an attempt to restore their youthfulness; the crude forerunner of dermabrasion or skin sanding.

We all remember the scraped knees of childhood. Several days after the fall, the scab came off to reveal fresh, pink and smooth skin. Living skin will always regenerate itself when its outer layers are shorn, either deliberately or accidentally. The technical difference between laser and chemical peel treatments is how the outer layers of skin are destroyed.

Lasers use a high-intensity, invisible beam of light energy that destroys superficial skin cells by boiling the water inside the cells. The treatment's strength is a function of intensity and length of time the beam is allowed to strike the skin. Lower power and shorter exposure time translates to less skin destruction and a shorter healing time, but a less profound result. Conversely, the deeper the damage to the skin, the more exuberant the healing process which generates the smoothest, tightest, most wrinkle free new skin.

Chemical peels achieve their result by a controlled chemical burn instigating the repair process. The spectrum of peeling agents or acids includes salicylic acid (a cousin of aspirin) at the weak end, and trichloroacetic acid (TCA) or phenol (carbolic acid) at the strong end. Phenol is considered by most sophisticated practitioners the most consistent, predictable and effective peeling agent. It is the agent preferred for deep peeling and creates the most impressive rejuvenation result.

PATIENT COMMENTARY

It's not quite a month since I had my chemical peel done, and already I am used to my remarkably younger face. People who know me either just stare at me or ask me straight out, 'What have you had done? You look great!'…People are astonished that a peel can do so much. Actually I was too. Although I've been in the medical field for twenty years, I did not realize that a face peel, under circumstances such as mine, could have far more effective results than a facelift. You were right. I would have been unhappy had I opted for a face lift, which would have left me with a tighter face but old skin. Thanks for doing a great job on my face, which now more closely resembles the young woman inside of me.

-Paula, marketing consultant, California

Some people show the signs of aging worse than others. Genetics plays a part. "Darker skinned people don't wrinkle as much as fair-skinned people, for example," according to Susan E. Downey, MD, Associate Professor of Clinical Surgery.

-USC Medical Journal

The ideal candidates for facial rejuvenation—either chemical or laser—are fair-complected with red or blond hair, green or blue eyes. Commonly, those of central or northern European ancestry. Because the process can cause some lightening or darkening of the skin, most skilled practitioners prefer to treat the entire face to assure uniformity of color. The area of facial treatment should "end" obscurely at the hairline and jawline to hide any potential minor color contrast with the adjacent untreated area. Therefore, a proposed treatment of only isolated areas or regions must be fully discussed during the consultation; there is the possibility of permanent, differential facial pigmentation.

I consider laser and chemical facial resurfacing rarely appropriate for acne scarring. Scar excisions and filling injections are generally better.

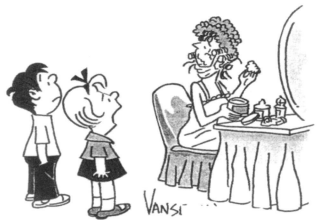

"Your wrinkle cream must be working, Mom.
You're getting a lot more of them."

The Challenge of New Technology

My personal observation is that laser technology never quite lived up to the dazzling promises for three prime reasons:

> The attention media gives to new procedures exerts a tacit but very real pressure on plastic surgeons to "conform," and this pressure may affect clinical judgment.
>
> -National Plastic Surgery Survey journal *Plastic and Reconstructive Surgery*, October 2000

● The unanticipated, high-dollar cost of keeping up with constantly evolving technology. The August 1999 issue of *Cosmetic Surgery Times* listed 20 corporations marketing 66 different lasers to physicians. How does one choose?

● The physician's "learning curve" was longer and more challenging than manufacturers claimed.

- The corps of laser providers—plastic surgeons, dermatologists, ophthalmologists, head and neck surgeons—was huge. The individual practice experience was diluted; not enough doctors could have a large enough patient volume for each to master the technique. Outcomes suffered.

- Patients treated in the first wave of enthusiasm were sometimes disappointed and even harmed. Let's briefly explore each of these observations. The nature of technology is dynamic. Immediately following the introduction of the carbon dioxide laser there was a rapid proliferation of different lasers. "Newer" and "better" lasers were parallel-marketed to the medical community, and to the public. Witnessing exciting segments on *60 Minutes* or *Dateline,* patients were demanding "the latest laser." But such high-tech equipment is never cheap, some costing over $150,000. It becomes a business issue. To afford that machine, a physician must treat a large number of patients. This creates a moral dilemma for the doctor: "How do I get the necessary experience quickly to become comfortable and proficient in this new technology without recruiting patients?" Yet, how can I pay for this expensive machine without a volume of patients?" An unsettling *Catch-22.*

> **A dilemma for the physician is whether to continue buying the newer technology at considerable expense or to wait for the "ultimate" procedure. Increasingly informed and discerning consumers force us to adopt newer technologies as competition and advertising make them aware of "better" ways to imrove their appearance.**
>
> **-Cynthia Weinstein, MD,**
> *Aesthetic Surgery Journal*
> January/February 1999

This brings us to the learning curve associated with laser technology. While the didactic, lecture-based weekend course is a bona fide component of continuing medical education, particularly for non-surgeons, new cosmetic surgical procedures require long-term follow-up, study, and evaluation to understand what really happens, to judge the result. Are there complications, problems, disappointments or dissatisfaction? So how does the beginner, now in practice (beyond classroom and laboratory and operating training), start performing a new procedure using unfamiliar technology? Yes, the doctor can take the laser manufacturer's course and practice on tomatoes, but one day he will be operating on a living, breathing human. And, yes, the company will happily send a technician to shadow the doctor during those first procedures and advise what settings—on his machine—are best for the patient's skin color, thickness, and degree of wrinkling. While this is a valuable service, it's only to get you jump-started.

INSIDER'S INSIGHT

Who's Teaching Doctors New Technologies?

New and Certified Pre-Owned Equipment

Lasers Intense Pulsed Light, Microdermabraders and more! Name the brand, we've got it — ESC Coherent, Parisian, PowerPeel, Propeel, top name a few! Save up to 70%! All devices certified with a comprehensive 40-point quality inspection. Training and warranties available. To learn about the newest trends in cosmetic and aesthetic services —photo Facial, Botox, Hair and Vein Therapy, etc. — Call us or email...

This ad in a recent plastic surgery newsletter underscores how equipment manufacturers' and dealers' marketing has become a subliminal force in continuing education for practicing physicians. Besides selling any and all equipment, the advertiser offers "training and warranties." Are the warranties issued on the training? Should equipment manufacturers supplant practicing MDs and university professors as our teachers? Who taught the manuafacturers what to teach and how to teach? Is there now a blurring between the continuing education of physicians and marketing of products and equipment to them?

This concerns me because I, too, need the services of medical professionals.

-RK

Having been a "student" in such situations, I would liken it to your first bicycle lesson: your dad holds onto the bicycle for support and stability, until you're peddling fast enough to gain speed. He then "let's go." You're now on your own!

The laser procedure itself is only the first step. Aftercare is just as important; if well done, prospects for success are increased. If aftercare is poor, the chance of problems, complications and disappointments increase. The technician rarely suffers through this phase, only the novice surgeon. Without seeing the patient's skin three, six or twelve months later, how can our visiting technical friend know the consequences of the treatment session's dial-setting?

Medical science is never 100-percent predictable. Results vary, even with the same mechanized "settings," because humans vary. The "art" of medicine is a combination of skill, knowledge, judgment, experience, and follow-up, without which our learning is incomplete.

Just as the novice practitioner and his machine move closer to perfecting an art form, the innovative laser industry delivers its "latest, super-improved model" that now must be studied, invested in, implemented and then mastered all over again.

Frankly, I believe lasers have been a bit oversold. Both to the "I-must-have-the-latest-laser-treatment" patient, and to driven, ambitious medical practices. I have my own substantial experience to draw upon. If laser wrinkle removal were more successful, more long lasting, less prone to problems and complications, it would be my number one choice. In my hands, lasers haven't done the job that phenol peeling has. Observation, long-term patient reports, and published laboratory studies—from multiple sources—suggest that deep phenol peeling will give a smoother, longer lasting result because of its deeper penetration. That's why I like it.

> No matter how accomplished, surgeons trying something new got worse before they got better, and the learning curve proved longer, and was affected by a far more complicated range of factors, than anyone had realized.
>
> Atul Gawande, MD
> "Annals of Medicine, The Learning Curve"
> *New Yorker*, January 28, 2002

Phenol chemical peeling, in my practice, is a constant. I don't alter the technique except for very minor variations based on scientific reports. There is no chemical peel industry tantalizing me with "newer models." If patients seek predictability in cosmetic procedures—as I believe they should—it seems reasonable that the process with a 40-year record of consistent performance, the "gold standard," should carry more weight than a newer technique with a limited history.

NEWER is not always better.

There's No Animal Lab for Testing New Cosmetic Procedures— We Humans Must Be the Guinea Pigs

Coronary artery bypass, hip replacement and heart transplants are some of modern surgery's spectacular triumphs. All were developed just during my professional lifetime. Before being brought to hospital operating rooms, they were tested and perfected in university laboratories and veterinary operating rooms. The techniques had to be proven feasible there before being used on humans.

Not so in cosmetic surgery. While all of us learned and relearned anatomy on human cadavers, new procedures, techniques, and technology can only be tried on living humans. And that is what makes it difficult to bring major change to my specialty. It *does not* and *cannot* happen overnight.

When some creative type at a medical meeting proclaims, "I have a brand new way to do a nose job—through the forehead," or whatever, not every cosmetic surgeon (thankfully) will discard his current, proven, comfortable technique the next day. In cosmetic surgery, change should evolve. Innovation must be slow, deliberate, and cautious. Perhaps only one step at a time. The "new and better method" must be tested, evaluated, retested, and examined. We must put just a toe into the water first.

I share this with you to curb your enthusiasm. To modulate your tendency to demand "that new technique" from your cosmetic surgeon minutes after seeing one successful case shown off on Fox News or CNN. Cosmetic surgery science should be cautious and deliberate. Mindful of risk to you, the patient. No swashbuckling here.

When a new idea, concept or technique is put forth, doctors must be skeptical. We need to protect you from its uncertainties and its possible side effects and complications. "Not working" would be bad enough, but what if it leaves you looking worse? How pleased will you be then? You will care much less that you are one of the first to have the procedure than the fact that it made you regret the decision to have it. Now I am not against progress, change or evolution. But, medical practice—cosmetic or otherwise—must be governed by that three-word Latin phrase—learned in medical school—that rules our professional conduct: *Primum No Nocere.* First, do no harm.

The burden in our specialty is particularly heavy because we cannot practice laser peels on monkeys, face lifts on dogs, or breast augmentation on pigs. Humans are our laboratories—for better or worse. We cannot hide our faults and failures. *Who said cosmetic surgery was easy?*

PATIENT COMMENTARY

Two years ago, I saw Dr. Kotler regarding a phenol peel. After much deliberation, I opted to have another doctor perform what appeared to be a less invasive procedure that promised to yield the same results, a laser peel.

The results of the laser peel were less than satisfactory for me. Although my cheeks and eye area were improved, the lines around my mouth did not improve at all.

The following year I returned to Dr. Kotler and consented to the phenol peel he originally recommended.

The results are phenomenal. No more lines. The lines around my mouth are gone, this even though I've been a smoker for many years.

I am delighted. I love my new face!

*-Carol, speech and educational therapist,
California*

Specific Questions to Ask if You Are Considering Non-surgical Facial Rejuvenation:

- What is the difference between a chemical peel and a laser peel? Which is better for me?

- Is it true not everyone is a satisfactory candidate for this procedure? How do I know if I am a good candidate? Is there a test to see if my skin is appropriate?

- Is there any special skin preparation necessary? Are there any products or medications I should *not* be placing onto my face prior to the procedure?

- Is it better to have the procedure done at a relatively young age, such as the forties? Or should I wait until the wrinkles are "really bad" in the sixties or seventies?

- What about my wrinkled neck? Can it be peeled or lasered too?

- Can facial surgery be done at the same time as chemical peeling or laser?

- Are all parts of the face treated? What are the pros and cons of treating all the face or sections of the face?

- Can blotchiness occur? If so, what can be done?

- Is it true you can never go back into the sun after this procedure?

- Will resurfacing the skin cause permanent lightening of my natural color?

- What will I look like during recovery?

- When can I wear makeup again?

- How long do these procedures last? Is it true that smoking, drinking, and other poor health habits will shorten the improvement life span?

> **Laser skin resurfacing decreased 14 percent between 1998 and 2000.**
>
> **-American Society of Plastic Surgery National Statistics, 2001**

Combination Of Surgical And Non-Surgical Facial Techniques

Many women over fifty-five, depending upon heredity and lifestyle factors are plagued by both "sagging" tissue and wrinkled skin. The sagging tends to occur earliest at the jawline, upper neck and under the eyes. Wrinkling may be most evident near the eyes, between the eyebrows, and around the lip and mouth areas.

PATIENT COMMENTARY

I will be 55 next month and everyone in this one stoplight town is amazed that I even got invited to my first baby shower in 20 years because the waitress who is having the baby assumed I was in my late 30s. When I tell them about the facelift and peel, they are fascinated. That kind of thing is rare in these parts. I have explained that in California, it's an unofficial law that you have to get things 'done' to stay looking as good as you can for as long as you can.

-April, screenwriter and chili manufacturer,
Tennessee

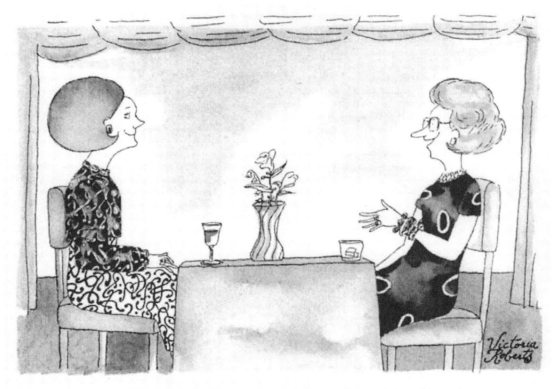

"Not only do you look marvelous but all of you looks the same age."

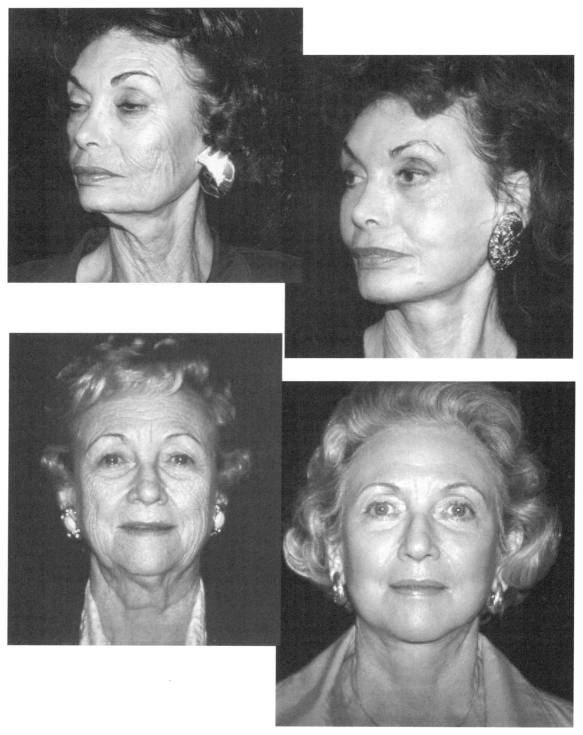

A combination eyelid lift, face and neck lift and chemical skin peel for both of these ladies was ideal. Surgery alone would have been disappointing.

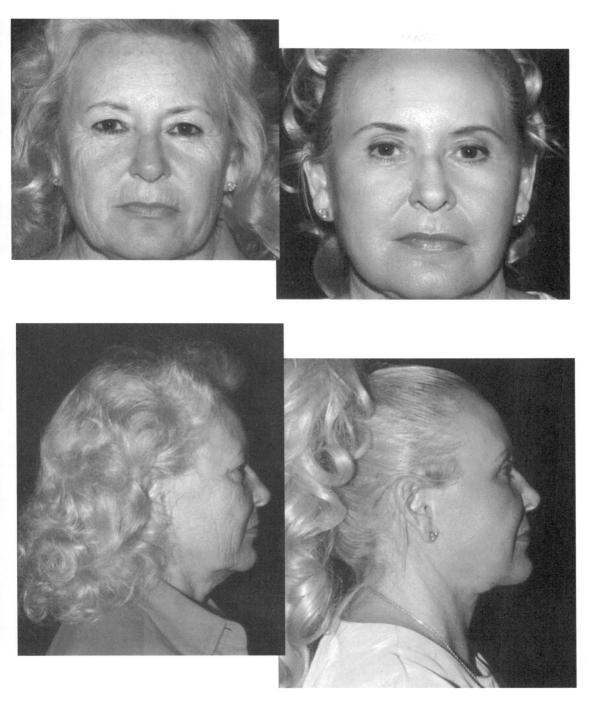

Eyelid lift, face and neck lift, chemical peel. When Darlene's husband saw her results, he scheduled a consultation. See his photos on page 113.

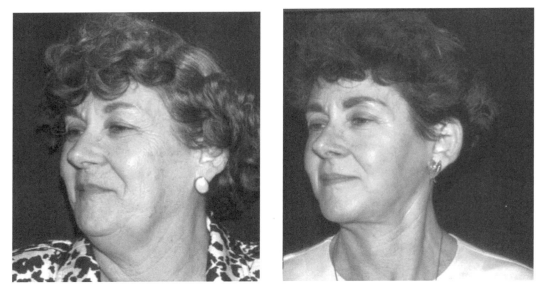

Chemical peel then weight loss, then face and neck lift—a winning program.

Because wrinkled and age-spotted skin must be addressed by a facial rejuvenation process, and sagging tissue must be corrected surgically, some patients require two different techniques to best enhance their appearance. Often a sequential combination of procedures—both surgical and non-surgical—is used. The result always exceeds that of any single procedure.

The good news is that each technique is effective and reliable; the bad news is that they cannot always be safely performed at the same session. Depending on which procedures are needed, an appropriate interval may be several weeks to three months. Usually, but not always, surgery is done first since the chemical or laser process may help further erase the nearly invisible surgical scars. The discussion about the ideal order of procedures and the interval between them must occur on an individual basis, at consultation.

FOREHEAD AND EYEBROW LIFTING
(Browplasty)

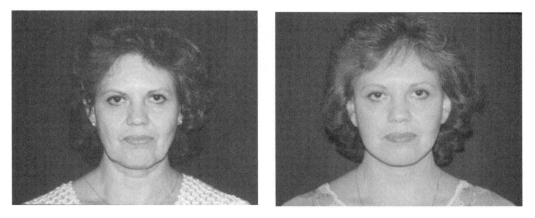

Forehead and brow lift plus face and necklift

As men and women age, their eyebrows may droop, creating a somewhat sad or oppressed look. Such sagging may coexist or be independent of other signs of facial aging. Correction of the forehead and brow may be done concurrently with any of the other surgical procedures described in this chapter.

There are alternative surgical solutions with different approaches and techniques. If tissues between the brows (just above the nose) and the eyebrows themselves have sagged to the same level, a forehead lift is indicated. Forehead/brow lifting yields a more natural, brighter appearance by elevating and tightening the eyebrows, forehead skin and muscles. In certain instances, frown lines and forehead creases also mildly improve. Results are best when brows are elevated to a "natural" level. Overdoing this procedure will create a very unsatisfactory "always surprised" look. This result should be avoided, since it cannot easily be corrected.

One route to the forehead and brow can be via a long horizontal incision at the hairline or paralleling it further back, depending on forehead height and scalp hair density. The second route is by "tunneling" under the scalp, usually through three short, hidden incisions. An endoscope (a tubular, lighted, periscope-like device) guides long-shafted microsurgical instruments to the target area to perform the necessary maneuvers. Technically, it is similar to knee and shoulder arthroscopy or colonoscopy.

Some surgeons perform a "temporal lift" that attacks only an outer, lateral (towards the ear) eyebrow droop. That technique is performed through an incision at or behind the temple hairline, above the ear. For some carefully selected patients, the outer, lateral drooping brows can be lifted by a direct approach, at the upper edge of the brows.

The decision regarding which procedure is best for you is made at consultation. With either surgery, healing is generally rapid and uncomplicated, and the patient can resume normal activities within one week.

Which Forehead/Brow Lift Technique is "Best?" Here are some conclusions regarding this important issue, from a recent medical paper:

> **We conclude that both endoscopic and coronal/pretichial (at the hairline) forehead lifts provide for comparable elevation at 1-year follow-up. Brow elevation in coronal/pretrichial forehead lifts may be temporary.**
>
> **-Steven H. Dayan, MD,**
> **"The Forehead Lift: Endoscopic Versus Coronal Approaches,"**
> **_Aesthetic Plastic Surgery_,   August 2000**

Specific Questions to Ask When Considering A Forehead or Brow Lift:

- What is the difference between "endoscopic" forehead brow lift and older techniques? Describe the "older" procedure. Why is the newer one better? With the "endoscopic" technique, where are the incisions made?

- My biggest problems are the deep lines between my eyes from frowning. Will forehead or eyebrow lifting help my appearance?

- My brows hang so low that they seem to cause problems with my vision. Does this mean both the brows and eyelids must be lifted?

- Is there a chance the nerves to the forehead can be injured? If so, what will I look like? Can this be repaired?

- Will there be a lot of bruising around the eyes and forehead?

- How soon can I return to work and normal activities?

NASAL SURGERY
(Rhinoplasty)

In the before and after examples, look for subtle but effective changes in nose and lip angle; the gentle raising of the tip; the slight lowering of the profile; subtle narrowing of the tip.

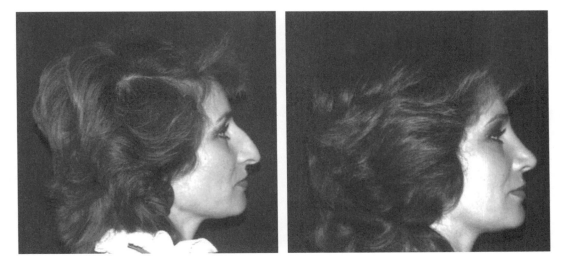

*Nasal surgery for an ethnic patient created
a natural unoperated look.*

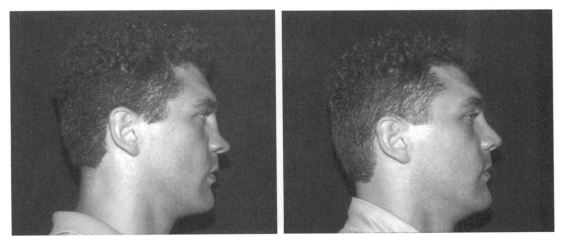

Nasal surgery corrected a major sports injury.

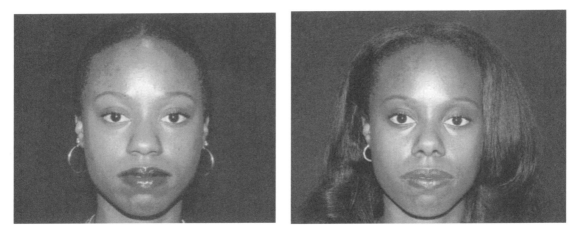

This attractive young black lady wanted refinement — not radical change.

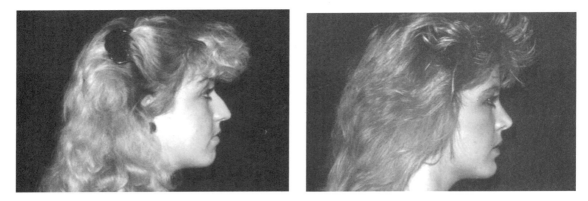

Chin augmentation enhanced the effect of this patient's nasal surgery.

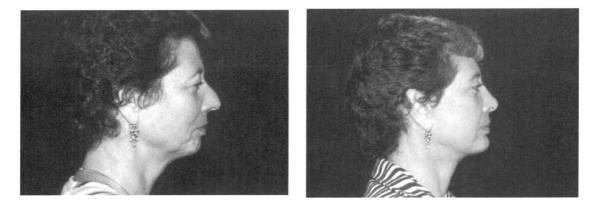

Nasal surgery and chin augmentation, face and neck lift, plus eyelid surgery created a very dramatic, yet natural-appearing improvement.

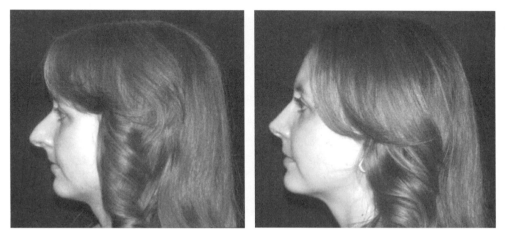

*The hump has been reduced and the entire nose recessed
(brought closer to the face).*

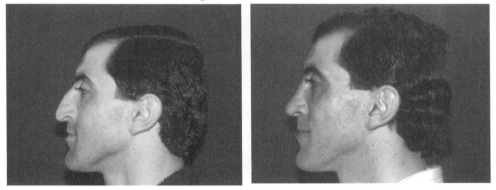

For gentlemen, the nose must not be overdone.

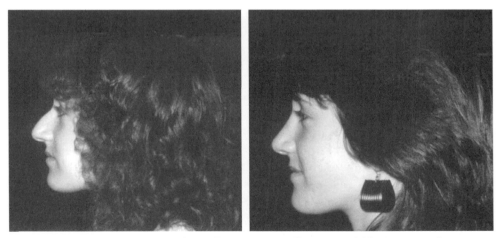

This young patient is rather tall so a very small nose would be inappropriate.

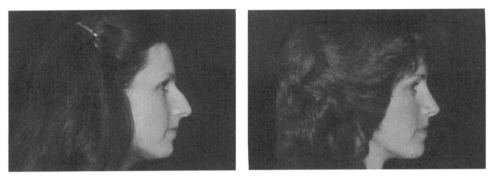

The nose was made smaller by raising the tip (shortening), removing the bump, lengthening the upper lip at the expense of the nose. The end result must harmonize with other facial features.

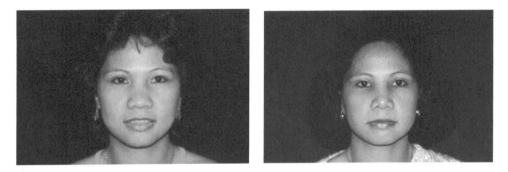

Cosmetic surgery for an Asian-American. The nose has been narrowed, the nostrils made smaller. The bridge has been raised using a solid plastic implant.

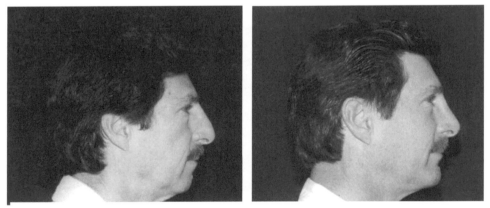

Nose and chin surgery dramatically improved this gentleman's appearance.

PATIENT COMMENTARY

It has been over a month now since I had my surgery and I just wanted to write to tell you how much I appreciate everything you have done for me. I cannot explain to you (although I'm sure many other people have said that before) how happy I am with the outcome. At first I wasn't sure what to expect, but now that the swelling has gone down, I really can say that I love it.

It is very rare to find people that listen to others. You heard exactly what my concerns were and you knew exactly what I wanted. The reason I know this is because you gave me the nose I have always wanted and the very nose that I asked you for. You and your staff made me feel so comfortable about the decision I had made and it made the entire process that much easier.

It has been so great to get such extraordinary feedback from my family and friends and to hear them all use the word "natural" in their responses. Some people didn't even notice it when they first saw me, and after I reminded them, they couldn't believe how NATURAL and beautiful it looked— which as we all know is exactly what I wanted.

Not only do I feel good but I feel freer. My breathing is immaculate and I just feel better. I can't thank you enough for your concern, care and patience. You made this decision one that I will never regret.

Thank you, thank you, thank you,

-Jaime, college freshman

A generation ago, most surgeons created the identical cookie-cutter, nose at every operation, with little regard for the individual patient's facial features. Invariably, the results were quite artificial looking and certainly unacceptable by current high standards. Today's taste calls for less radical change and a nose that does not appear to have undergone surgery. The surgeon's highest compliment is remaining incognito.

When you can spot an obvious "nose job," two failures took place. The second failure was that of the surgeon: an inability—conceptually or technically to create that individualized, unoperated-appearing, natural nose. But the first failure, the primary cause, was that of the patient: poor surgeon selection. Perhaps homework was not done, questions were left unasked, or before and after photos were either ignored or not requested. An overdone, too-pinched, too-scooped unnatural nose is the product of an inadequately trained doctor working on an unsuspecting patient. Perhaps the patient was content with the sign on the door that said, "Plastic Surgery" or "Cosmetic Surgery" and assumed the doctor behind the door was good at every cosmetic surgery procedure. Now you know better.

> **Successful nasal cosmetic surgery is brain surgery. You change the way the patient sees himself; you change a life.**
>
> **-Howard Diamond, MD nasal surgeon extraordinaire, New York City**

Ideally, a nose should look natural, well proportioned to the face and so pleasing that it calls little attention to itself. Unsatisfactory outcomes tend to be "overdone." Too upturned, too ski-sloped, with overly prominent nostrils, or a "pinched" tip, or an overall unnatural or artificial look.

PATIENT COMMENTARY

I am writing to let you know how happy I am with my new nose. It has been six months and I still love it…

Once the initial swelling went down, I could tell it looked 100 percent better than before. Your instructions from me were " I still want my nose; just a better version of it." The best part is that friends that I had seen only the week prior to surgery couldn't tell I had had it done. They commented only how well I looked, and asked me if I cut my hair. The new and improved version of my nose looked so natural.

The inside work you performed, however, was much harder for me to immediately gauge. It seemed like I was breathing better but I wasn't sure of the full difference and benefit, until the L.A. fires. I didn't recognize just how much better I was breathing until all those noses around me that suffer with allergies, as mine used to do, became stopped up; mine didn't…but it wasn't until everybody started sounding very nasally and rummaging through my desk for nasal decongestants did I realize the difference. I have not had a stuffed up nose from an allergy attack since the surgery. Also, I have not needed to use a single dose of nasal decongestant since. This is saying a lot, since I used to buy Drixoral six boxes at a time. Even when I recently had a head cold, my nose only became a little stuffed up by comparison to what I am now used to. What I call a stuffed up nose now is better than what used to be a good breathing day before the surgery.

When it comes to allergy symptoms, ability to breath and general appearance…I guess I would say, "I won by a nose."

-Valerie, businesswoman, California

PATIENT COMMENTARY

I want to thank you for the wonderful job you did on my nose. Not only is it tailored to my facial features, but to my personality as well. One of my biggest concerns when I was choosing a doctor was that all of the noses on all of the patients looked exactly the same. It was as if the doctors I had spoken with had found one nose that worked and had simply chosen to reproduce it over and over again without regard to the individual. When I went through all of the photos and watched the video in your office, I thought, "Finally, a doctor who doesn't mass produce his looks."

-Heidi, student, California

No Such Thing As An Easy Nose Job

Let me now share a special little secret: even some of the most sophisticated, cosmetic surgeons shy away from performing some very difficult nasal cases, particularly "redos." They wisely refer such cases to colleagues who major in nasal surgery. Why? Because they are smart enough to recognize that the "nose job" is technically the most difficult procedure in cosmetic surgery. It is both functionally and conceptually complex when compared to other cosmetic procedures of the face and body.

Nasal surgery takes unusual manual dexterity and superior eye/hand coordination. The operation is usually done entirely through the nostrils (although some surgeons use the "open rhinoplasty" approach combining both internal and external incisions). In either case, nasal surgery is a challenging prospect even for the most sophisticated surgeon. All architectural changes are made inside after tunneling under the skin of the nose. Typically, tissue is removed to make the nose smaller, but sometimes natural tissue—or a plastic part—is added to strengthen the tip or raise the bridge of the nose. Doing all this through the nostrils is like operating through a keyhole. Custom, miniaturized surgical instruments perform sophisticated techniques and maneuvers. An eighth of an inch, more or less, can make a difference in appearance. Placing and tying stitches is challenging (the good news for you is that those stitches dissolve). As a resident-trainee, at first it took me over two hours to perform a routine nasal surgery. And it was not much fun. Too hard. Today, the same operation takes a mere 45 minutes; now I enjoy it.

> **The most popular cosmetic surgical procedure among men was nose reshaping with 150, 185 performed.**
>
> **-American Society of Plastic Surgeons National Statistics, 2001**

In many nasal cases, the surgeon faces the daunting task of not only creating a better looking nose, but also improving nasal airflow, straightening if crooked (very challenging), reducing sinus problems, and improving allergy symptoms. The objective of this total overhaul is a nose that looks good and works well. A big order.

Why am I providing this additional, technical information on nasal procedures in this chapter? Because if there is such a thing as a super-superspecialist, then a top nose surgeon is it. Even some terrific cosmetic surgeons will deliberate over accepting some nose cases: But that's O.K. As specialized as we may be, we all can't do everything equally well.

> **Twenty percent of men would like to change the shape or size of their noses.**
>
> **-Men's Health**

Having Cosmetic Nasal Surgery—Trouble Breathing, Snoring, Sinus Problems? Why Not Take Care Of Everything At One time?

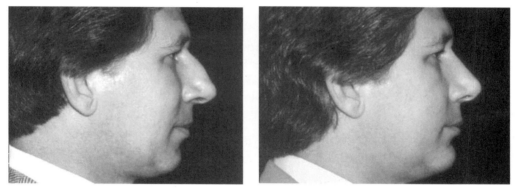

His wife brought him in so she could sleep better. He was happy she did; he breathes well and looks good.

If you are planning to have nasal surgery, be sure to ask yourself if you are comfortable with your breathing. Or, perhaps you snore or have been told you have a "sinus problem." If you suspect you have one of these problems and want to do something about it, this is the best time. Consider doing both cosmetic and functional nasal surgery together. Here are several smart reasons:

- One pre-operative physical, one set of laboratory tests.

- One anesthetic. Why "go under" twice?

- Same recovery time: five to seven days. Same time off work.

- You will save money.

A complete cosmetic nasal surgery consultation should automatically include questions about your breathing and an examination of the inside of your nose to evaluate the nasal anatomy, the airflow and status of the sinuses.

The Top Three Male Procedures In 2000

- **Nasal surgery**
- **Eyelid surgery**
- **Liposuction**

-The American Society of Plastic Surgeons, *Annual Report 2001*

Cosmetic surgeons who have that special expertise in nasal surgery are also trained to manage breathing issues on the inside of the nose as well as appearance issues on the outside. Many of them, as part of their residency, were trained by ear, nose and throat specialists who are the masters of the nose and sinuses.

Regardless of whether or not you recognize that you have a breathing problem, the surgeon needs to determine your airway status—before surgery. Here is why:

- The patient who has a minor breathing problem may not be aware of it—until after cosmetic surgery—when he will be more attuned to the nose's function. The surgeon should recognize the diminished airflow *before* the procedure so that the patient does not mistakenly attribute any breathing difficulty—temporary or permanent—to the cosmetic surgery. The breathing baseline must be established first.

- If the outside is crooked, most often so is the inside with negative implications for breathing. Straightening the nose for cosmetic purposes entails straightening the inside to achieve the goal. The surgeon will tell you that he must do the inside to optimize the outside and that your breathing will benefit. A bonus.

- The value in recognizing how well you breathe—before surgery—is that the examination is a wake-up call. If you ever wondered about how your breathing can be improved, here is the time to learn. Then you can make your decision before surgery. And, some people—who have only known inadequate breathing—do not realize they could *breathe better* if something was done. They have no idea what normal good breathing is like because they have never experienced it. A specific office exam—using only a nasal spray—can demonstrate how well you could breathe after surgery.

What are the common reasons for blocked nasal passages that cause poor breathing and might be responsible for "sinus problems" and possibly snoring?

- **Deviated septum.** The vertical, internal partition that separates the left and right nasal passages may be deviated (not midline but crooked). The problem is commonly secondary to an injury—recognized or unrecognized; it is quite common in male athletes.

- **Enlarged turbinates**. There are three within each nasal passage. Each is a shelf-like projection of bone covered wih the same skin-like membrane that lines the entire nose. The turbinates' corrugated configuration cleverly increases the internal nasal surface area amplifying the three unique functions of the nasal passges: to warm, humidify and filter incoming air en route to the lungs. Turbinates can contribute to obstruction either because they are unnaturally large or the membrane-cover swells and thickens because of allergy, pollution or other factors.

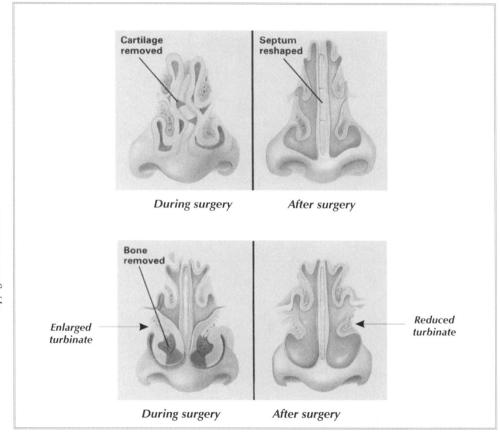

Nasal septoplasty and turbinate resections. The classic operation to reverse blockage and improve air flow.

Most people burdened with a blocked nose have it because of a combination of both septum and turbinate abnormalities. The ideal operation corrects both problems simultaneously. The crooked septum, constructed of bone cartilage, is straighten and the bends and buckles which narrow the passages are removed. The two lower, or inferior turbinates, normally the biggest and also most prone to abnormal enlargement, are reduced in size by a variety of means. Each surgeon has his favorite combination of techniques; by any means the success rate is extremely high. These procedures are well established and reliable; some were perfected over 75 years ago.

Such coring out of the obstructed passageways translates to a big rush of air flow and increased patient comfort because we know that airflow is raised *exponentially* (the 4th power for you physics fans) to an increase in the diameter of the passage through the nose and into the sinuses which may be likened to internal rooms or chambers that open into the nasal hallway. Sinus problems—headaches, pressure and thick tenacious mucous drainage—occur when the nasal hallway is blocked. Air cannot get into the rooms until the hallway is cleared.

NIGHT BLIGHT
The Burden of the Unfortunate Who Sleep With
Those Whose Noses Are Blocked

The bad thing about a snorer
In fact, the very worst,
Is, with two people in the room
He always drops off first.

Snoring—a very common problem—may be relieved as the airflow is once again allowed to pass through the nose. A blocked nose reroutes incoming air to pass through the mouth—nature's second choice and a weak pinch hitter. This is what creates the noisy, inefficient breathing we call snoring (when the floppy soft palate is forced to vibrate).

More good news. Regarding cost issues, two factors favor combining the cosmetic and functional procedures. The first is that the total cost is always less than having two components done as separate procedures. For those with health insurance, there are usually policy benefits for the internal functional surgery to improve the airway which is a medical issue. If you wish to invoke your insurance benefits, this will call for some interaction between you and your insurance company, as well as between your surgeon and the insurance company. See **Chapter 6, "About Fees,"** where the subject of insurance coverage of functional surgery is discussed in detail. Patients will realize an economy benefit from having the functional surgery done at the same time as the cosmetic surgery. Then, much of the basic setup costs or "overhead" including operating room time, anesthesia services , medications and supplies are apportioned to the functional procedures. Hence, the obligation of the insurance company. In such cases the charges for the cosmetic portion become an extra, add-on charge, since the surgeon is "already there."

Insurance or no insurance, if you are having cosmetic nasal surgery and you are not happy with your breathing, or not even sure if you have a problem, discuss it at consultation and ask the surgeon if he feels it is wise to combine procedures; you save time and money, and minimize anesthesia. Makes sense.

Nose Jobs For Senior Citizens

"I always wanted to have my nose done…sorry I didn't do it when I was younger."

"I wanted to do my nose, but my family was not supportive."

"As I get older, I could swear my nose is growing!"

"Thanks for suggesting I fix my nose with the other procedures. I thought about it often, but it was never a priority."

Having heard these comments consistently throughout my many years of practice, I realized that positive change at any age is priceless. In fact, piggybacking nasal surgery onto a face-lift or eyelid surgery is an ideal add-on.

- Nasal surgery adds only twenty to thirty minutes additional operating time.

- Recovery is the same.

- Lifting the drooping nasal tip and/or removing a bump are youth-producing maneuvers that perfectly accompany other procedures.

- Incremental expense usually reflects a 50-70 percent discount when done in conjunction with other procedures.

While the patient typically focuses on the more overt signs of aging: baggy eyelids, sagging neck, heavy jowls, and wrinkled skin, cosmetic surgeons are trained to see the whole picture. Many times the doctor will raise the subject of complementary procedures that will enhance the overall results. The choice however is always the patient's.

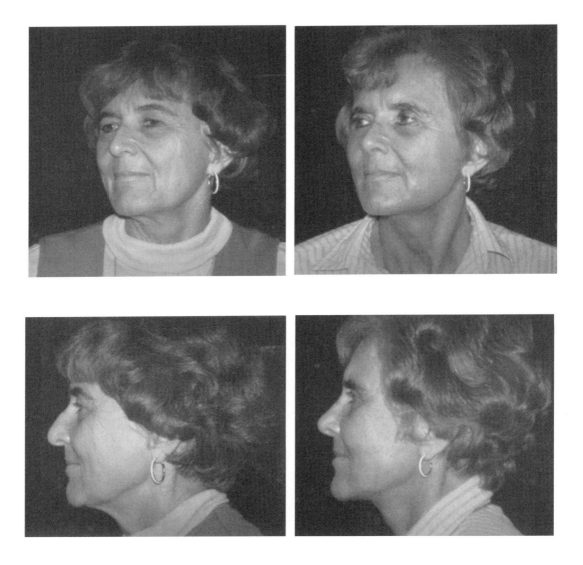

Rhinoplasty — always conservatively done, can be an excellent youth-producing auxillary procedure for patient having a face and neck lift.

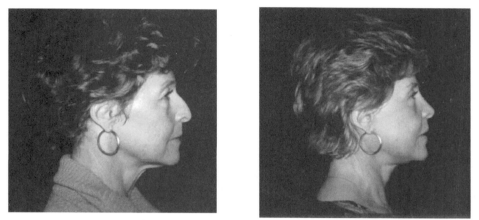

Rhinoplasty and neck and face lift do wonders.

PATIENT COMMENTARY

> *I'd like to tell you that I always remember you every time I see my nose in a photograph. People say it looks very natural and would never imagine I had plastic surgery. I consider it the best compliment for me, and of course, for the good job you did.*
>
> *-Olivia, international flight attendant*
> *Rome, Italy*

Specific Questions to Ask When Considering Cosmetic Nasal Surgery:

- What parts of my nose need attention? Describe my new nose.

- Can you assure me that the nose will look "natural"? Why do some "nose jobs" look unnatural?

- Will you have to break my nose?

- Will I have incisions hidden within my nose, or an external incision between nostrils? Why?

- If the nose is made smaller, what happens to the extra skin? Is it cut out?

"Yes, I've been trying to hold on to every element of my youth," says Faye Wattleton, head of the Center for Gender Equality. "I don't think there's anything wrong with that. If we can retard the process of aging, the quality of life is improved because aging does bring certain changes."

from *Don't Count the Candles Just Keep the Fire Lit!* by Joan Rivers

When I smile my nose comes down and nearly meets my lip. Can that be corrected? How? Will it affect my lip?

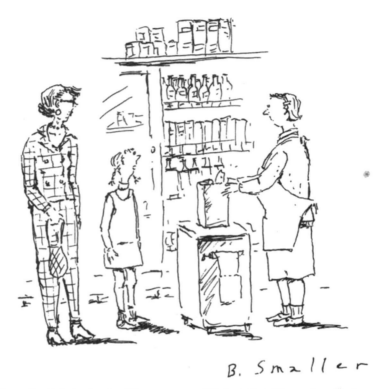

"Actually, I do look a lot like my mom. It's just that I have her first nose."

What is the earliest age at which cosmetic nasal surgery can be performed?

Is it true that the nose grows as people get older? What can be done about that?

Can I combine nasal surgery with other cosmetic facial surgery?

I want to have my breathing improved at the same time. Can this be done? My health insurance will cover the breathing portion of the operation. Does having cosmetic surgery at the same time along with it present a problem to my insurance company?

● What is the difference in recovery if both the breathing operation and a cosmetic procedure are done concurrently? I understand "packing" is put in the nose. How long does it stay? Is the packing different for breathing improvement?

● How long before the swelling goes down and I look decent?

● When can I resume normal activities? Apply make-up?

● Can a too-small nose be made larger?

● I have broken capillaries on my nose? Does that mean I can or cannot have nasal surgery?

NECK SCULPTURE
(Submentoplasty)

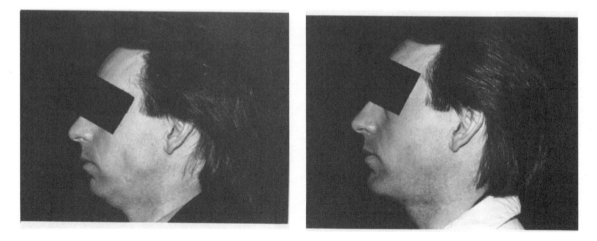

Chin augmentation and neck sculpture improve appearance.

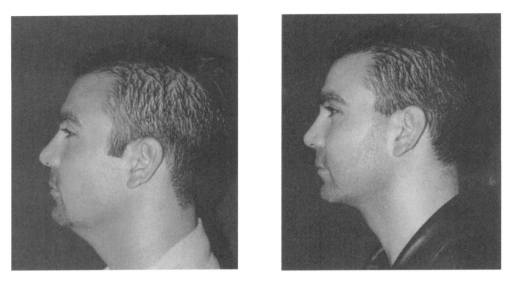

Neck scupture is appropriate to remove fat that fails to disappear with weight loss.

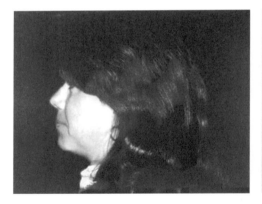
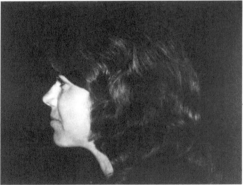

Before

After

Neck sculpture

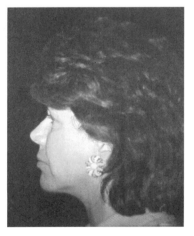

After 20 years it still looks good!

Neck sculpture optimizes the definition between chin and neck by removing excess fat beneath the skin and, as needed, tightening of the sagging platysma neck muscle. Its success is dependent upon the neck skin having enough elasticity to retract and redrape satisfactorily after sculpturing. Like a new, tight rubber band, rather than an old, used, stretched-out one.

PATIENT COMMENTARY

> *The lift you gave to my neck and to my life will hold me forever grateful to you. Just four weeks after my surgery, I met the man of my dreams and we'll be walking down the aisle very soon. Perhaps the way I felt about my 'new' self did the trick.*
>
> *-Barbara, teacher, California*

This procedure is most appropriate for younger patients who have inherited a "double chin" or for those patients who, despite reasonable weight loss, retain a neckline that is still poorly defined. Though not a substitute for the more ambitious face and neck lifting, neck sculpturing may indeed delay the day of more extensive procedures since it addresses the area that is frequently the first to demonstrate aging.

The entire procedure is done through a fine, horizontal, hidden incision just below the chin. No skin is removed—only fat— and, as indicated, excess flabby muscle. Frequently, liposuction alone is used through one of several shorter incisions to sculpt the neck most efficiently. Some surgeons use a slim suction/drain tube that automatically and painlessly withdraws fluid after surgery; this device reduces swelling and bruising. The tube is removed after one to two days.

Should a chin implant also be desired, it can be inserted through the same incision. The coexistence of a receding chin and a poorly defined neckline is not infrequent. In such cases, combining procedures delivers an optimal result.

Specific Questions to Ask if You Are Considering Neck Sculpturing:

- Is this the procedure used for a younger person who has a "double chin"? Should I try diet and exercise first?

- What do you actually do in this operation? Do you liposuction to remove fat? Do you tighten any muscles?

- I am young but have a hanging neck muscle. What can you do about that? Why does elasticity count? If my skin is not taut, is it true that this operation is not appropriate?

- How is neck sculpturing different from the neck portion of a face and neck lift?

- If I have a chin implant, how does it affect the overall surgery and my recovery?

- Are drains put in? For how long? Where do they exit? How are they removed? Will it be painful?

- How soon can I resume normal activities?

- What will happen if I gain or lose substantial weight after the procedure is done?

Hopefully this procedure-by-procedure guide gave you valuable insight into the range of cosmetic surgery options available to you and tips on what to look for as you evaluate prospective surgeons and their work. It should also prove handy in asking the right questions. Your preparation will help eliminate incorrect assumptions, unrealistic expectations, and misconceptions about the procedure(s) you are considering.

Beware The "Latest" Or "Newest" Procedure

Cosmetic surgeons—like all people in science—like to be part of progress: new techniques and innovative procedures. We are tinkerers and fixers by nature.

Medical meetings and conventions wow attendees with the latest high technology, new operations, improved drugs, and clever instruments. Every month, medical journals, are laden with "a new way to do…" or imaginative innovations. The march towards perfection never stops, nor should it.

For some patients, ostensibly the beneficiaries of this progress, the rewards may not always be gratifying. Here's why: everything "new" has to have the kinks worked out. Often, this takes months or years. You may have been told never to buy a car in the first-model year. Do you want to be part of the "test population"? A cosmetic surgery purchase is permanent. It cannot be returned for a store credit or refund. Because surgical changes are irreversible, you must weigh the benefits versus the risks of any procedure. But the dilemma—for the patient and doctor—with a new operation, technique, or procedure is that no one knows yet the balance between risk and reward. To do so, one would need the following information:

> **The rapid advances in medical technology always bring mixed blessings. On the one hand newer technology often allows us to achieve better and more predictable results. On the other hand, it forces us to continuously learn new procedures just when we are becoming comfortable with the more established techniques. This alone is difficult enough, not to mention expensive when considering the capital outlay on newer equipment.**
>
> **-Cynthia Weinstein, MD,**
> **Aesthetic Surgery Journal**
> **January/February 1999**

- The percentage of success or failure.

- The nature and percentage of complications.

- The longevity: how long will the procedure last?

- Unforeseen problems and disappointments. As a patient, it is easier to "sign up" for a time-tested procedure for which the above answers are well established.

Personally, and because of my innate Midwestern conservatism—born, raised and schooled in Illinois and Wisconsin—I tend not to be the "first kid on the block" to offer the so-called "latest and greatest" to the patient sitting before me at the consultation. I put myself into the shoes of the patient and ask whether I would want to have a minimally-proven, as yet uncertain, procedure performed upon me. It may well prove to be more unpredictable and less successful than an existing, well-established, "tried and true" operation. And remember, we are unlike the rest of the medical world. Medicine often faces failure of an established treatment program, (for cancer, for example). There, the use of an experimental and potentially life-saving new drug has little downside.

In cosmetic surgery, we are not desperate for miracles.

We Have Come A Long Way

I completed my residency and became a board certified specialist in 1973. Here are some of the procedures, products, and technologies unknown then:

- Liposuction.

- Laser skin resurfacing.

- Calf and pectoral implants.

- Endoscopic forehead and brow lifts.

- Cheek implants.

- Collagen injections.

- Botox.

- Safe, general anesthesia for cosmetic surgery performed as an outpatient, outside the hospital setting.

- Computerized monitoring in the operating room.

- Computer imaging.

- E-mail to transmit the computerized image to and from office and patient's home (see Computer Imaging, Chapter 5).

In 1973, there were no satellite dishes, cellular phones, DVDs, fax machines, personal computers, home VCRs or electric cars, either. The next 25 years should be even more interesting medically and otherwise.

What I don't want to hear is that you can't find the money for plastic surgery. If you can afford a trailer home, you can afford a face lift.

-Joan Rivers

7
ABOUT FEES

Secret: **High fees don't necessarily guarantee superior results. Low fees are not always a bargain.**

IF YOUR SELECTION OF A SURGEON IS DETERMINED PRIMARILY BY FEE—high or low— ultimately you may be disappointed with your choice. You cannot accurately judge a professional by fees alone. Each professional has variables that drive the fee schedule. For example:

- Office overhead. Rent, equipment, supplies.

- Number and quality of staff. The better the staff, the higher the salaries.

- The surgeon's expertise. Superspecialists are efficient surgeons. They require less (costly) operating room time. There's value in that.

- Other value-added items which factor into the fee can include:

  - Medications (prescription and non-prescription) and supplies. Are they included in the fee? Always ask.

  - Aftercare. Home nursing or recovery hide-away charges may or may not be included.

■   Patient transportation. Some practices provide limo service the day of surgery. This service may or may not be included in the fee.

But, high or low, you need to know exact numbers. No guesswork. So, as you consult and collect quotes, be sure you know exactly what services are—and are not—included.

INSIDER'S INSIGHT

Higher Fees For Lesser Talent?

There is solid logic in the fact that more specialized professionals command greater fees. They offer a higher level of service; they are compensated for the longer duration and higher expense of their advanced education and training. They are rewarded for their mastery.

Alternatively, there is no good reason to pay more for less expertise, skill, sophistication, and experience. But somehow, it happens everyday. People overpay for mediocre talent. The over-payers are usually those who either have money to burn or who did not bother to ask themselves why one doctor asked them to pay more than another. They did not do their homework. They did not ask enough good questions. There should be a reason for higher-than-average fees — and a good one.

-RK

In addition to the specifics of products and services rendered, there is the intangible: your general comfort level. Some factors that impact comfort can include:

●   Confidence that the doctor has the talent to surgically deliver what you expect.

> **Of all the products sold, of all the stores in the United States, none of the leaders are the cheapest brands.**
>
> **-Jay Levinson & Seth Godin**
> *Get What You Deserve*

●   Professional and attentive conduct during the consultation period. Does the surgeon listen carefully to your needs and desires? Does he express respect and appreciation for you as a patient?

●   Satisfaction that the surgeon's support staff is well trained and will assist in you in a caring and professional way.

●   Belief that the operating facility and after care service meet high standards for your safety and comfort.

- Acceptance of the fees as reasonable and affordable for the amount and quality of service performed.

- A healthy "gut feeling" about the entire undertaking.

> **The money I spent on my wives' cosmetic surgery was a lot more fun than the money I spent on their divorce lawyers.**
>
> -Otis, "professional" bowler, Wisconsin

If you feel satisfied that your surgeon and his staff meet these criteria, you will feel good about writing the check and should have an excellent experience.

Charges are a function of time expended on the patient's behalf by a team of highly skilled professionals. In addition to the surgeon, services are provided by nurses, aides and administrative staff members. Anesthesia is critical for your comfort and safety, so the anesthetist or anesthesiologist is another indispensable and valued part of the team. With four or more professionals in the operating room, and administrative staff members seen and unseen, you can appreciate the multiple services being rendered for the fee. Care is given before and after the operating room time; this routine "pre and postoperative care" should be included in the surgeon's fee.

- Expect separate charges for the surgical facility and anesthesia services. These sophisticated, licensed, certified surgical centers cost more to build, staff and operate than a small, single, operating room in a doctor's back office. Anesthesiologists (physican specialists), by virtue of their pedigree, rightly command higher fees than nurse anesthetists. These "costs of quality" impact charges. *Reminder: Know where you will be having surgery and who will be assisting.*

- The familiar real estate adage, "location, location, location" applies to your surgeon. It costs more to run a practice in Beverly Hills than it does in Oshkosh. The difference in real estate and labor costs will be reflected in doctors' fees. World-class, sophisticated medical communities with large teaching hospitals nearby are ideal professional environments. However, they are generally located in the higher rent areas of our biggest cities. *Reminder: Expect to pay more where top specialists congregate. Consider it another quality cost ... an investment.*

● You may find yourself paying (too much) for an interesting intangible: the practice's "image." A few cosmetic surgeons, seeking only wealthy patients, assume that the ultra-affluent view the purchase of cosmetic surgery services as they would the purchase of a luxury car or fine jewelry. But I maintain that this formula does not necessarily work in my industry. Paying more—without a good reason—gives you no assurance of a better outcome. Just look at Hollywood, where some misguided celebrities display unsatisfactory—and even tragic—results. Perhaps they also thought: "You get what you pay for." They bought into price, but did not hire quality: the superspecialist. *Reminder: You do not necessarily "get what you pay for" in the world of cosmetic surgery. Be sure your research can objectively justify higher -than-average fees.*

> **The bitterness of poor quality is remembered long after the sweetness of low price is forgotten.**

High Fee — Wrong Reason

A local veteran surgical nurse shared the following observations and insight with me:

> "Dr. A's fees are high—and for the wrong reason. His results are not above average, there's no justification there. He does not take on the toughest cases. His practice gives Chevrolet—not Cadillac—service; acceptable, average, but not great. His fees are high because he is very slow in the operating room. It takes him two hours to do a routine cosmetic nasal surgery that would take you 45 minutes. But in his mind, he is billing like a lawyer: hourly. So his fee is inappropriately high because the patient is overpaying for his inexperience and lack of expertise."

What you just read is very telling. And a very special bit of "insider information" that is important to share with you. Actually, I never thought of fee setting in the light that our veteran nurse just described. The very best surgeons I have seen are rarely "slow." They are not fast for speed's sake; it's that they are very efficient and waste no time. They do not spend five minutes walking around the table and looking at the nose and trying to decide what to do. The "A" surgeons already have a plan. They know what to do even before they walk into the operating room. They deliberate in advance. Then they operate without hesitation or uncertainty.

Efficiency is critical because after a certain amount of time elapses, the local anesthetic wears off, bleeding increases, and swelling becomes burdensome. The hapless, inadequate surgeon is now "drowning in the case" and has very little chance of coming up for air. It is very disturbing to see these amateurs struggling against odds that only worsen minute-by-minute.

Every time our nurses talk about assisting in a four-hour nose job, or a five-hour eyelid surgery, or a ten-hour face lift, I shudder. I know they were teamed up with an inexperienced, inefficient, amateur surgeon who probably should not be doing these cosmetic procedures. Because the patient will be—at least—disappointed and, possibly, even endangered.

INSIDER 'S INSIGHT

There may be a good reason for you to pay a surgeon a fee that is 10 to 25 percent above average. But, double or triple? Okay, I guess, if you can't think of another way to spend money.

-RK

Same Operation — Why Different Fees?

Now that you understand the financial basics, you will want to know how to compare professional fees. Let's take a common scenario experienced by patients while comparison-shopping: A prospective patient consults with Dr. A, who recommends a facelift and whose office provides a fee quotation of X dollars as an all-inclusive fee. At the next consultation, Dr. B tells the same patient he needs a facelift but Dr. B's facelift is 50 percent higher than Dr. A's. The patient is rightfully confused. How to reconcile the difference in charges!

Comparing professional fees is not easy; never "apples to apples." Cosmetic surgery is an art form, each surgeon an artist. No two cosmetic surgeons do the same operation identically. Regardless of the artistic variations, procedure-specific, technical variables will effect the fee.

An example:

● Dr. A's "facelift" may differ greatly from Dr. B's. Not all facelifts are identical. One doctor's procedure may include an aggressive neck sculpture technique while another's focuses on the forehead and brows with less attention to the jaw and neckline. There may be major qualitative differences in similarly titled procedures. Does the facelift include neck surgery? Are eyelids upper and/or lower, included? *Reminder: Know the components of the procedure the surgeon is quoting.*

There can be quantitative differences as well. Dr. A's preferred "neck sculpting" or "neck lifting," to improve a sagging or "double chin," may involve only superficial liposuction through a tiny incision or incisions. Dr. B's neck work may include, in addition to the superficial liposuction, removal of the deeper layer of fat as well as tightening of the lax platysma neck muscle that causes those vertical bands running from the chin to the mid or lower neck. This platysmaplasty, an additional step creating an internal "corset," further defines the neck and jaw line. But this more ambitious neck surgery requires a longer (but still hidden) incision, and many more maneuvers. So while both Dr. A and Dr. B name their procedures identically, Dr. B's method adds additional time and complexity compared to the lesser procedure. But, Dr. B's result will probably be superior and apt to last longer. Expect, therefore, B's fee to be higher. *Reminder: Understand the objective of the procedures the doctor recommends. Be sure you understand how the doctor intends to accomplish the mission. If you are unclear, request more information including drawings that you can understand. And take notes! Be studious!*

PATIENT COMMENTARY

I spent all this money tailoring my clothes. There is no reason why I couldn't do the same for my face.

-Elinor, designer
California

ROBERT KOTLER, MD, FACS

Patient Name:_____ Surgery Date:_____Today's Date_____

Procedure: _____

_____

Fee Quotation - Cosmetic Surgery

Procedure Fee:	$_____
Outpatient Surgicenter Fee:	$_____
Anesthesiologists Fee:	$_____
Total	$_____

Sample Fee Quotation Sheet

After you've gathered several quotes, if you can't adequately rationalize or understand the fee differential, consider the following advice: all things being equal, a mid-range fee is most likely consistent with good value. A "low" fee may signify a lesser procedure, be reflective of lesser levels of facility or anesthesiology services, or in some cases, alert you to an inexperienced surgeon anxious to build a cosmetic surgery practice—not on ability, but on low fees. The "high end" fee quotation may come from a practice where the surgeon is deliberately marketing his services to the super-rich, or where the practice prefers to serve fewer patients, but at a higher charge per patient in order to maintain its income.

Why Payment in Advance?

This insures that the patient has the resources to provide for the services, that scheduling the surgery is not done casually, and that the surgeon's commitment is matched by the patient's.

What If You Need A "Touch-Up"?

Most cosmetic surgeons do not charge for "revision" or touch-up surgery. Surgeons are paid on an all-inclusive, per-case basis. In contrast, surgical facilities and anesthesia professionals charge by the hour, like attorneys, accountants, and consultants.

Here is a reasonable and common practice with respect to these touch-ups:

- If the treatment required is minor and can be done in the surgeon's office treatment room, there is usually no charge.

- If a return visit to the operating room at the hospital, surgery center, or office O.R. is required, a minimal charge for the operating facility and for the anesthesia specialist is proper. The charges should be discussed and "a fixed fee"—without any add-ons afterwards—should be agreed upon.

- The best time to understand all financial responsibilities is before surgery, at the consultation. Be sure to ask if your surgeon includes touch-ups in his fee. And also ask about possible additional charges by the surgical facility and anesthesia specialist.

- The top practices tell you their business practices—in writing, up front—because nobody likes surprises "afterwards."

"What About Insurance?"

Although health insurance does not cover purely cosmetic surgery, there are insurance benefits available for some reconstructive procedures that typically may overlap a cosmetic procedure. Services that improve function or that are necessary to repair the damage done by an injury or tumor are covered. For example, if one's upper eyelids are so heavy and redundant that vision is impaired, some or all of the procedure costs may be a covered benefit. If one's nose was deformed by an accident—causing breathing or possibly sinus problems—then benefits for the functional correction of the internal passages, and/or reconstruction of the damaged exterior, may be covered.

If you believe that insurance may be applicable to your condition, the examining doctor will need to file a report with the insurance company including his finding and proposed treatment. The insurance company will evaluate this report and advise you and your surgeon whether or not the proposed procedure is covered. The doctor's office may be required to provide additional documentation to the insurance company—photographs, x-rays and consultant's notes—before the insurer grants a "go ahead" or "precertification."* Whether the insurance company writes a check will depend upon yet

---

* Make sure you receive this official permission from insurer, in writing, before your surgery.

another record review *after* your surgery. Because of the unreliability of today's insurance carriers, most practitioners must ask you to pay for the proposed service—in part or in whole—prior to the procedure. When the insurance company pays, you will be reimbursed the amount of deposit which you made prior to the surgery.

INSIDER'S INSIGHT

Please Do Not Ask A Doctor To Cheat

Every specialist who performs nasal cosmetic surgery has been asked, at least once, to "bill my insurance." That translates to "bill the insurance for a functional, insurance-eligible procedure, even though that's not what was performed." Perform a rhinoplasty, (cosmetic, and hence not covered by insurance), but bill the insurance carrier for a septoplasty (an internal, functional operation — not cosmetic — to open the air passages).

You are, in effect, asking a licensed professional to commit fraud. For a doctor to accept this risk could mean loss of license and criminal prosecution after investing half a lifetime training and building a practice. You would be an equal partner in that fraud.

Thankfully, only a tiny percentage of doctors participate in fraud. Eventually, they are all caught and bring shame to themselves and their families, and discredit to their profession. A doctor without integrity not only cheats insurers, he may also cheat patients. Patients should consider if this is the person into whose hands they would place not only their nose, but their lives.

-RK

Medicine is an occupation that strives to maintain trust. In the heart of every patient there must dwell the questions: Can I trust this doctor? Is he/she committed to excellence? Does he/she care about me?

-R. Scott Jones MD, FACS
Presidential Address to
The American College Of Surgeons, April 2001

If I were two-faced, would I be wearing this one?
                                        -Abraham Lincoln

8

LOCATION
Considerations

Secret: Your Choice of Operating Facility Can Be As
              Important As Your Choice Of Surgeon.

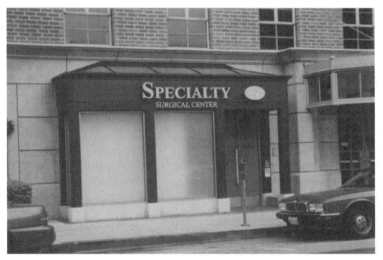

*A licensed, fully-accredited outpatient surgery center in a medical building
is an excellent choice for surgery.*

Hospital, Doctor's Surgical Suite or
Outpatient Surgery Center?

FOR OVER THIRTY YEARS, MUCH COSMETIC SURGERY HAS
BEEN PERFORMED AS AN OUTPATIENT SERVICE; that is, "in
and out" the same day, no overnight hospitalization required.
You may wonder what difference location makes if you are there for
only a few hours. Based upon your medical history, the procedure(s)

to be performed, other practical considerations, your doctor will recommend a facility. It will serve you best in terms of comfort and safety for you, and efficiency and risk reduction for the surgeon. A doctor must anticipate any problems that could arise, and he must be confident of having access to the people and equipment necessary to make your surgery successful and complication-free.

The Important Safety Standards of Accredited Surgical Facilities

- **MD supervision of anesthetic services.**
- **Pre-operative medical assessment by a physician or super-vised non-physician.**
- **Adequate physical plant. This includes operating room size, hall lighting, availability of oxygen, suction.**
- **Basic equipment including oxygen and blood pressure mon-itor, ventilation machine.**
- **Emergency drugs, supplies and equipment.**
- **Staff trained and credentialed in Advanced Cardiac Life Support.**
- **Back up oxygen and electricity systems.**
- **A hospital-type, post-anesthetic (recovery) unit.**

- "Managing Your O.R.: Clarification of Anesthesia Standards and Guidelines"
Aesthetic Surgery Journal,
November/December 2001

During 2000, the American Society of Plastic Surgeons noted that 37 percent of cosmetic procedures were performed in offices, 28 percent in hospitals and 35 percent in outpatient surgery centers. Regardless of where your procedure takes place, you should be aware of certain key standards of excellence and safety. Several national organizations provide the guidelines.

- Most—though not all—hospitals in the United States are accredited by the Joint Commission on Accreditation of Health Organizations, (JCAHO). Sponsored by the American Medical Association, the American College of Physicians, the American College of Surgeons, and the American Hospital Association, JCAHO visits and evaluates the

> **The survey showed that patients prefer outpatient to inpatient surgery and that they prefer ASCs (ambulatory or outpatient surgery centers) over hospitals. They cited less paperwork, lower cost, convenient location, parking, less waiting and the friendly staff.**
>
> *-Outpatient Surgery Magazine,*
> **Special Edition,**
> **January 2002**

hospitals to determine if current standards are being met. A hospital found "in compliance" is recognized as "accredited." Such accreditation must be renewed on a regular basis. Should your doctor plan to perform your procedure in a hospital, you should ask: "Is the hospital accredited by the Joint Commission?"

● Ambulatory surgicenters and office facilities should have identical standards of excellence. Here, too, there are organizations that establish high standards. Most prominent among these are the Accreditation Association for Ambulatory Health Care (AAAHC), the Joint Commission for Accreditation of Health Organizations, (JCAHO), and the American Association for the Accreditation of Ambulatory Surgical Facilities (AAAASF).

If the ambulatory surgery center caters to a large number of elderly patients, it may also seek Medicare certification from the federal government.

● Licensure by the state health department is another credential held by many outpatient surgery centers. Such licensure denotes the meeting of state-approved standards that match those of licensed hospitals. If the facility in which your surgeon intends to perform your procedure is Medicare-certified and/or state licensed, you can be comfortable that safety and care standards have met hospital standards.

Assuming a level playing field of equal accreditation, let's explore the pros and cons of hospitals, surgery centers and doctors' offices for cosmetic surgery:

Hospitals as a Location Choice

Unless you have a medical condition warranting hospital level service, or are a patient under the age of fourteen (only hospitals are expected to have medications and equipment suitable for all ages), a hospital may not be your best choice. They are generally large and impersonal. They are expensive, and more importantly, rarely focus on or specialize in cosmetic surgery. Today's hospitals are overtaxed by staff shortages and tight budgets. Their mission is to serve the needs of sick patients. The consequence is that cosmetic surgery patients are rarely treated in the attentive and comforting manner they expect.

Doctor Surgical Suites

Assuming they are duly licensed, certified or accredited, and thus meet the strict requirements of safety outlined above, doctors' office surgical suites can be adequate and appropriate for cosmetic surgery. Optimally, the facility should be in a medical campus building because it is important to have other doctors available in case of emergency. At the least, there must be a nurse anesthetist or physician-anesthesiologist on the surgical team. Charges for office facilities tend to be far less than hospitals and somewhat less than outpatient surgery centers.

It's safe to say that outpatient surgery today is more technologically advanced, faster, and less invasive than ever. Nevertheless, we are facing a crisis in one of the most rapidly growing segments of outpatient surgery—those cases performed in physician office-based settings. As the number of procedures performed in these facilities grows (more than 9,000,000 cases were done last year, which is more than the number of procedures performed in ambulatory surgery centers), morbidity and mortality rates continue to be unacceptably high.

The horror stories abound—from the case of ophthalmologists who lost a patient while attempting to simultaneously administer anesthesia and perform an elective cosmetic procedure, to the 24 deaths that occurred in office-based cosmetic surgery suites in Florida, prompting a now-notorious moratorium on office-based surgery. In virtually every one of these cases, the standard of care was compromised—either the practitioner or ancillary personnel were not qualified, or they weren't prepared for emergencies, or there wasn't enough staff on hand.

The good news is that several national associations, including the Accreditation Association for Ambulatory Health Care and the Joint Commission for the Accreditation of Healthcare Organizations, have already put together common-sense guidelines to ensure patient safety and high quality of care in all ambulatory surgery settings. In my own office-based anesthesia practice, we voluntarily underwent Accreditation by the AAAHC. The process, while not easy, was not overly cumbersome or expensive, and going through the experience made us a better, safer practice.

The bad news is that in most states the accreditation process is voluntary for office-surgery facilities. To date, only one state—California—has mandated accreditation for these facilities, and only one specialty organization—the American Society of Plastic Surgeons—has required its members to accredit their facilities or risk losing membership.

Some state governments have attempted to jump on the regulation bandwagon by either forming their own regulations or adopting already-established guidelines, but they've done so in a haphazard, disorganized manner, without appropriate input from any of the various medical societies or hospitals, ambulatory surgery center, or nursing associations.

-from "A Call To Action" by David Barinholtz, MD, anesthesiologist in *Outpatient Surgery*, January 2002

PATIENT COMMENTARY

This note is to thank you all for the wonderful treatment I received before, during and after my recent nasal surgery.

I really like the idea of a surgery center located within your facility rather than a cold, impersonal hospital where costs are escalated and the service leaves something to be desired. Everyone in the center was highly efficient, professional and friendly; they definitely made me feel more at ease than I would have at a hospital. No time was wasted; the entire procedure took only four hours from the time I walked in the door until I was ready to go home. There was always someone there to answer my questions and put me at ease.

Thank you for making the entire process a very pleasant, memorable experience.

-Kerry, administrator
California

Outpatient Surgery Centers

These are appropriate for nearly all cosmetic surgery procedures and are particularly suited for cosmetic procedures. Unlike hospitals, surgery centers offer niche or boutique services that can be exquisitely specialized. Since they typically have two to four operating rooms, there is usually plenty of capable support staff, a critical issue should there be any emergency. Nurses, surgeons and anesthesia specialists are on site at all times. Surgery centers are best located in buildings devoted to medical services, or on a medical campus. Both provide safe, seasoned, secure places for medical procedures, and professional environments for pre- and post-operation consultations.

> **Ambulatory Surgery Center— Not A New Concept**
>
> **The first modern multispecialty Ambulatory Surgery Center opened in 1970 in Phoenix, Arizona. The proprietors were anesthesiologists Wallace A. Reed, MD and John L. Ford, MD.**
>
> *-Outpatient Surgery,*
> **Special Edition, January 2001 Outpatient Surgery Centers**

Most importantly, surgery centers offer the patient privacy and anonymity in a tranquil, relaxed atmosphere. Fees are typically somewhere between those charged by a hospital and an office suite set-up for outpatient procedures.

Firsthand Experience With Outpatient Surgery Centers

In the 1990s, I was involved with a state-licensed, U.S. Government certified, outpatient surgery center. I participated in its design and served as Medical Director (chief quality control officer). This private, two-operating room center, located on the ground floor of a major medical building in the heart of Beverly Hills' "Doctors Row," had a perfect safety record in its eight years of operation. Nearly 10,000 procedures were performed with NO significant complications. No deaths. No cardiac arrests. Only four patients transferred to a local hospital for observation and all four were discharged the next day. The secret of this successful run?

- **Hand picked, top quality, professional staff.** The surgeons were highly specialized and experienced. Most held university teaching positions. Staff privileges were given by invitation only and acceptance was predicated on meeting tight standards. Nurses were equally specialized. In the operating room, the surgical assistants were super-specialists. Many had been assisting in cosmetic surgery exclusively for over twenty years. The recovery room was staffed with Registered Nurses (RNs) familiar with the demands of intensive care and cardiac care, and had experience treating problems during surgery or recovery.

● **A safe facility.** This center was designed by architects and space planners who limit their work to medical facilities; they don't design houses, warehouses or office buildings. The center was built to the high standards necessary for state licensure and government certification. The facility employed specialized consultants for management and quality assurance programs. It was not easy to build and operate a quality, safe, outpatient surgery center; there is no more tightly regulated business. But that's why you—as a patient—want to have your surgery performed in a similar credentialed, safe, surgery center; it has passed all the tests.

● **Doctor-anesthesiologists only.** Our anesthesiologists were all superspecialists with deep experience in cosmetic surgery, and that they dedicated to the facility and its mission of excellence. They did little hospital work, primarily outpatient cosmetic procedures. They had the right personalities for this field: warm, friendly and caring. Professionals who took time to make the patients feel comfortable and confident. And that's what set them apart from the average.

Traveling for Cosmetic Surgery

> **We had such a good time in America. At the moment, we are very busy but remember you every morning when we get up and look into the mirror.**
>
> **-Angelika, Kornelia, and Silvia**
> **Munich, Germany**

In our mobile, global society it is important to address traveling for cosmetic surgery. Some people travel within the United States, some come to the USA from foreign countries, and some Americans go abroad.

Southern California has long been considered a Mecca for cosmetic surgery. People throughout the United States and beyond our borders make the journey to Southern California, and particularly Beverly Hills, for surgery. The most common reasons cited include "highest safety standards," "the most sophisticated treatments," "best surgeons." Indeed for many foreigners, cosmetic surgery's art form is not as advanced in their homeland as it is in the United States.

While some "immigrate" for cosmetic surgery, some Americans "emigrate." Recently, *The New York Times* published a catchy article about Americans combining foreign travel and cosmetic surgery. Our specialty has long been aware of this, but rarely has it been seen as news. What makes it newsworthy is that several countries, hungry for American dollars, are waging an aggressive marketing campaign to attract Americans seeking low-cost cosmetic surgery. No question surgery costs less in Mexico, Costa Rica, Brazil, Thailand or Russia. We have had a little peek into this world from patients and prospective patients who have shared their experience or that of a friend with "foreign cosmetic surgery." Some are happy. Some are disappointed. For you, if you consider this option, the dilemma lies in the "what if?" "What if" there's a serious complication or unintended results? What is the contingency plan? What happens when you're 10,000 miles from home?

Medical Tourists

Number of Out of State Procedures and Reasons Patients Give:

- **60% Lack of qualified physicians in their area**
- **43% Comfortable vacation-like recovery**
- **28% Cost**
- **20% Referral**
- **16% Reputation**

-from *The 2000 Survey*,
American Academy of Facial Plastic and Reconstructive Surgery
June 2001

In the U.S., we have very stringent licensure and credentialing processes for doctors, hospitals, outpatient surgery center, clinics, etc. No other countries match our standards. This should concern you. In a third world country, proper sterilization techniques, safety of the blood supply, and available, competent emergency care cannot be taken for granted. Most third world countries have nowhere near the safety standards, modern equipment, or highly specialized personnel to which we've grown accustomed.

There is some excellent work performed by foreign cosmetic surgeons (some American-trained) who are operating in their homeland. There are also some patients who receive terribly botched surgery and must then return home for an American surgeon to do the necessary repair work. Certainly this double dose of surgery will erase any savings.

> These days, there are plenty of people in Thailand—from government officials to hotel owners to doctors and nurses—banking on the country's new status as an international capital of discount plastic surgery...'Have the surgery and see beautiful Thailand—get it?'...Most American plastic surgeons take a dim view...Follow-up visits are a problem, they point out, and cultural ideals of beauty differ—and more importantly—so do medical credentials and standards of care. 'All the best plastic surgeons in those countries come to the U.S. to train. So why would an American go there for surgery?' said Daniel Morello, MD, president of the American Society for Aesthetic Plastic Surgery.
>
> - "Nip, Tuck and Frequent-Flier Miles",
> *The New York Times,* May 6, 2001

This is not to say problems and complications never occur in Beverly Hills, New York or Miami. But, consider the world-class medical back- up available here in the United States, if needed. As one patient commented, " I do not turn over my face—and potentially my life—to the low bidder 8,000 miles from home." If you want to visit an exotic locale, take a vacation. If you want cosmetic surgery, be cautious and analytical in your decision making.

8 Wise Questions For Americans Emigrating for Cosmetic Surgery

1. When I arrive, where will the consultation be and at what time?

2. Who performs the physical exam to assure my health is satisfactory for the operation(s) and anesthetic?

3. What if my desires are inappropriate and surgery cannot be done safely or satisfactory?

4. If I opt for the surgery, will there be a board-certified doctor-anesthesiologist in attendance at all times?

5. What if I don't feel comfortable with the surgeon, the anesthesiologist, or the facility?

6. Can I get my money back and fly home without reper- cussion?

7.   Who will care for me immediately after surgery?

8.   What if something happens after my return home? Who manages the problem? Who pays?

If you need medical attention, get it in the United States. We have the best trained medical personnel and finest equipment anywhere.

Diana Rosen, author *American Pride*

The surgeon was discussing a forthcoming operation with a wealthy patient. "Would you prefer a local anesthetic?" he inquired.

"I can afford the best," replied the wealthy patient. "Get something imported."

- Jacob Braude, author
Braude's Treasury of Wit and Humor

9
ANESTHESIA—Who is "at the Controls"?

Secret: Know the difference between an anesthesiologist and an anesthetist. Only one is a doctor.

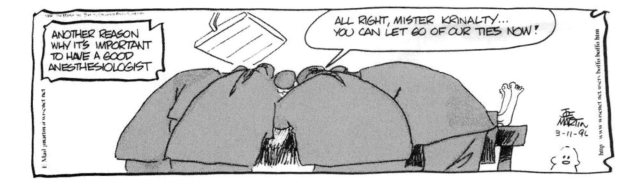

An Important Date In Anesthesia History

Last evening, as we were informed by a gentleman who witnessed the operation, an ulcerated tooth was extracted from the mouth of an individual without giving the slightest pain. He was put into a kind of sleep, by inhaling a preparation, the effects of which lasted for about three-quarters of a minute, just long enough to extract a tooth.

– from a notice that appeared in the *Boston Daily Journal* on October 1, 1846[*]

ANESTHESIA IN SOME FORM IS REQUIRED FOR ALL COSMETIC SURGERY PROCEDURES. What you may find surprising however, is the relative importance of the relationship between the type of anesthesia used and who is at the controls.

There are three modes of anesthesia your surgeon will consider:

● Local anesthesia, injected by the surgeon

● Local anesthesia with intravenous sedation

● General anesthesia. The patient is unconscious; vital signs are constantly monitored.

The Length And Type of Procedure Will Dictate The Choice of Anesthesia

Local anesthesia, in which the patient is fully awake, is appropriate for only the most minor procedures. For example, a surgeon might consider it for mole removal. Local anesthesia for cosmetic surgery is like having Novocaine® at the dentist: you are aware of the procedure but the area is numb; you feel no pain.

Local anesthesia with sedation can be safely used for many common cosmetic procedures. Sedatives, painkillers and tranquilizers are administered intravenously for immediate effect. This procedure is similar to having sodium pentothal or a similar sedative for dental surgery, such as a wisdom tooth extraction. You will be asleep, unaware of the surgery, and not remember or sense any of the

---

[*] The day after the first recognized administration of a general anesthetic by William Morton, DDS, a Boston dentist. Fifteen days later, on October 16, 1846 the first successful surgical procedure under general anesthesia was performed at the Massachusetts General Hospital.

procedure. A surgeon may consider this form of anesthesia for simple rhinoplasty, routine upper and lower eyelid surgery, or cosmetic correction of the ears.

INSIDER'S INSIGHT

How Safe Is General Anesthesia For Cosmetic Surgery?

Very safe. Statistics are available that should comfort you.

In a journal article published in January, 2001 the authors reported an eighteen-year study of over 23,000 procedures performed in an office-based, outpatient surgery center managed by doctor anesthesiologists. There were no deaths and no serious complications.

Having visited the reporting practice with its attached modern, properly equipped, accredited surgical facility, I was not surprised at its superb history.

This enviable safety record is not unique, but as you will learn in this chapter, it is the product of focus, dedication, diligence and a high degree of specialization.

-RK

General anesthesia, once reserved for inpatient hospital cases, has become more common in outpatient practices. Indeed, technological and drug advances developed in recent years have made general anesthesia the choice for longer, more intricate cosmetic procedures. High-tech monitoring devices that continuously report on vital signs and associated data, coupled with newer anesthetic drugs, have greatly improved the safety of general anesthesia. These innovations allow even the longest operations (up to seven or eight hours) to present little risk to the patient. Under general anesthesia you are put into a state of unconsciousness. Your vital signs are constantly monitored. Facelifts, necklifts and combination procedures would be examples of cosmetic surgeries requiring general anesthesia. In most cases, local anesthesia is injected into the operative site—after you are asleep—to reduce the depth of general anesthesia (for safety) and to reduce bleeding.

So, who is most qualified to administer anesthesia in each of the above scenarios? Who should be in control?

Local anesthesia, without sedatives—as in a dental office—is a low-risk technique and requires minimal electronic monitoring. This is only suitable for the least invasive procedures, as a scar "touch-up" or mole removal. Administration by the surgeon is appropriate.

Sedation-anesthesia (given intravenously for rapid onset), or **general anesthesia,** must be administered by an anesthesia specialist, not the surgeon. The surgeon's priority is dealing with the details of performing the procedure. He will be far too preoccupied to also be responsible for the administration of anesthetics. When potent pain medications, tranquilizers and sedatives are introduced into the body, observation, monitoring and management of vital functions is a full-time job.

Two different types of medical specialists are qualified to administer anesthesia: nurse anesthetists and doctor anesthesiologists. Nurse anesthetists officially work at the direction of the surgeon, but in practice, they perform their services independently. Nurse anesthetists are licensed registered nurses, who have pursued additional specialty training in anesthesia—the nursing parallel of a physician's residency.

> I can't say whether one needs an anesthesio-logist. I know when I seek care for my family or myself, I want the best-trained professional that is available. That will always be the anesthesiologist.
>
> -Barry L. Friedberg, MD, Clinical Instructor of Anesthesiology, University of Southern California, Los Angeles

Anesthesiologists are medical doctors who have trained a minimum of three years after medical school in their specialty, defined as "the practice of internal medicine in the operating and recovery rooms." The doctor-anesthesiologist is responsible for control of key internal organ functions, particularly those of the heart and lungs.

It is important that you are comfortable with the anesthesia issue. Most likely, your surgeon will have a consistent routine for each procedure performed, including the type of anesthesia employed. Most superspecialist cosmetic surgeons prefer to work with a small cadre of anesthesiologists. By working together they develop consistent patterns and systems that reduce the chance of error—much like a basketball team where each player can anticipate his teammates' moves. Safety levels rise with team consistency. This level of familiarity and stability is more difficult to achieve if a surgeon is teamed with a new anesthesiologist for each operation.

You should ask what type of anesthetic the surgeon prefers, whether the administrator of the anesthetic will be an RN (registered nurse) anesthetist or an MD (medical doctor) anesthesiologist, and how well the surgeon knows this individual. Understanding the difference in education and training will help shape your preference. Your choice should be honored.

Understandably, there is some "rivalry" between nurse-anesthetists and doctor-anesthesiologists.   Another medical turf battle. Read here the words of a doctor-anesthesiologist who, prior to becoming a physician, was a nurse-anesthetist. Her remarks were recently printed in the newsletter of The American Society of Anesthesiologists:

Can Nurse Anesthetists Replace Anesthesiologists? Only If They Become Doctors.

I was a nurse anesthetist for ten years. I was well trained; my academic performance and technical skills were significantly above average. I taught student nurse anesthetists and even directed a school of nurse anesthesia for a short while. Then I entered medical school. I did so with no interest in pursuing anesthesiology as a specialty. You see, I thought I knew everything there was to know about the administration of anesthesia. I was sure there would be a new, exciting and challenging career path beckoning brightly at the completion of my medical education.

My fourth year of medical school included a mandatory clinical rotation in anesthesiology: Ironically, I was assigned to the same hospital that had employed me as a nurse anesthetist. I knew nearly everyone, "This will be a snap," I thought. But it wasn't. Everything was familiar: an operating room I had worked in hundreds of times, equipment I had used. Then I was introduced to the patient. That patient was a completely different entity than the last patient I had anesthetized as a nurse anesthetist. It was as though I had always seen in black and white and suddenly had color vision! What an astonishingly complex and vulnerable being who was lying there! Why had I not appreciated this before? What had changed?

I had, of course. I was a fourth-year medical student who had been a nurse anesthetist. I had the mind of a doctor now. I had struggled and learned all about pathology, histology, anatomy, pharmacology, internal medicine and surgery. I had mastered the basics of physical examination, clinical diagnosis and treatment. A stethoscope was no longer just something to check lung sounds and heart rhythm: it was one of many diagnostic tools at my disposal. With it I could identify murmurs, extra heart sounds, rubs, fine rules versus coarse rules, and normal and abnormal bowel sounds. Under supervision and sometimes overwhelmingly critical observation, I had treated patients with hypertension, diabetes, heart disease, lung disease and neurologic conditions. I had a clear understanding of how difficult all this was and that the outcome of one's efforts could not be relied upon to be positive. So it was with this new perspective that I was viewing the patient lying before me in that operating room—and I was terrified. How little I really knew! How much there was to learn!

I applied and was accepted as an anesthesiology resident in the same university hospital setting that had awarded me my nursing degree. I anticipated being "ahead of the pack," for a bit, at the start of anesthesiology residency, confident that my technical skills would give me some advantage. That lasted about two weeks and then we were all on level ground again. I struggled along with everyone else for the rest of the three years. Now, I love being an anesthesiologist. I love the problem solving, the pharmacology, physics and physiology involved in every anesthetic. I thoroughly enjoy working closely with nurse anesthetists in a "team" setting that is defined by anesthesiologist supervision of nurse anesthetists.

Unfortunately, nurse anesthetists really do believe that they can do everything that an anesthesiologist can do, and do it better. I know I thought so. As a group, they mean well and I respect them enormously. But they have no idea how much they do not know. Nurses are not physicians. They cannot practice medicine. As nurses they require physician supervision.

So why remove the physician supervision requirement? The only answer I am aware of is that "anesthesia is safer now." Really? Do patients believe that anesthesia is so safe that it doesn't matter that a doctor may not be involved or have any responsibility for its administration?

I am one of the few who can see both sides of the issue clearly and, I hope, impartially. The nurse anesthetist who wants to be a doctor will have to do it the way I did—the hard way.

-Kay S. Rost, MD
Rochester, Minnesota

While the chance of a problem with anesthesia is miniscule, if a difficulty should arise, it could be catastrophic in the wrong hands. You should seek to reduce that risk to the lowest level possible. Decide whom you prefer to have administer you anesthetic. Make your feelings known, without equivocation to your doctor. It's your body. It's your life.

Now, Anesthesia Has Cosmetic Surgery Superspecialists!

The spectacular daily triumphs of coronary bypass, heart valve replacement, liver, kidney and joint replacement are not feasible without the astonishing capabilities of modern anesthesiology.

Anesthesiology has been a recognized physician specialty since the founding of the American Board of Anesthesiology in 1937.

In **Chapter 4—Why Superspecialization Is So Important**, you learned about *superspecialists.* Doctors, who by obtaining additional training beyond residency and board certification, practice only a narrow portion of their core specialty. Today, there exists analogous subspecialization and even superspecialization within anesthesiology also: subspecialty training in cardiovascular, pediatric, neurosurgical and obstetric anesthesiology. Also, available to fully trained anesthe- siologists are fellowships in pain management and critical care.

The subdivision of anesthesiology is a very positive trend for all patients and particularly cosmetic surgery patients. Office and outpatient surgery center anesthesia demands techniques and medications that differ from major, hospital in-patient surgery.

Here is why anesthesiologists are migrating to the office and surgery center world. They live in a distinct practice environment: short, elective surgery performed on healthy, low-risk patients. Also personally it is attractive—regular hours, freedom from night and weekend duty. And less stress than emergency and other unpredictictable hospital work. To provide continuing education for these subspecialists, there are three societies: the **Society of Ambulatory Anesthesia**, the **Society of Office-Based Anesthesiologists,** and the **American Society of Anesthesiologists.** Acceptance into these organizations is predicated upon demonstrated focus and experience in outpatient and office-based anesthesia respectively.

In our major cities, there is enough cosmetic surgery to allow some anesthesiologists to practice cosmetic surgery anesthesia exclusively. Anesthesia delivered by such superspecialists is ideal.

If you value the wisdom of selecting a superspecialist cosmetic surgeon, ask that doctor to select an anesthesiologist who is as specialized as he is. By doing so, you further enhance the prospect for having a safe, comfortable and positive anesthesia experience.

Appreciation for the review of the above section on anesthesia superspecialists to Shawn Taheri, MD, board-certified anesthesiologist and Medical Director of the Summit Surgical Center, Beverly Hills.

I had my nose done and I never told my husband, and now I'm pregnant and I'm afraid that the baby will be born with my old nose and my husband won't know where it came from. P.S. I destroyed most of my pictures, so he's never seen me with my old nose.

-Amy, quoted in "Tales From the Front,"
Chicago Tribune

10
AFTERCARE

Secret: Complications can occur after "the last stitch." To reduce that chance know your doctor's philosophy on aftercare.

As important as what to do, say the surgeons, are the things that one should be meticulous about avoiding. "It all boils down to wound healing," says Manhattan plastic surgeon Z. Paul Lorence. The highly competitive plastic-surgery community might bicker over techniques and bragging rights, but when it comes to stating the worst offenses that can be committed against a healing face, it is unanimous: smoking and exposure to the sun. "We would never recommend that a facelift patient go to St. Bart's," Lorence says. "If you do so, you're likely to return with a raised and glistening scar."

As for smoking, some doctors, including Beverly Hills plastic surgeon Robert Kotler, are now refusing to operate on patients who won't give up nicotine. "I just can't do it," he says. "There is no question that the smoker has done irreparable damage to the skin and the blood vessels; the complication rate is too high." Kotler warns that a patient who resumes her nicotine habit shortly after surgery is also doing herself a great disservice. "Because smoking worsens the blood supply," he says, "the skin can break down and form another scar."

-from "Well Healed"
by Patricia Reynoso
in *W*, November 2001

Since hospitalization is rare in cosmetic surgery, you must anticipate where you will recuperate, who will take care of you and what to expect. The superior practice provides excellent care before, during and after your surgery. Also, knowing your options and being familiar with common post surgical experiences should alleviate anxiety.

Where Do You Stay?

Some patients will be most comfortable convalescing at home. This can be appropriate after nearly all cosmetic procedures if there is either a responsible adult available and willing or, better yet, a trained medical professional present. Professionals who do "home care" are available anywhere. They may be registered nurses, practical nurses or medical assistants. Since there is no major nursing duty involved in routine cosmetic postoperative care, their title and credentials are less important than their cosmetic surgery experience level. The professional in attendance should be familiar with the procedure's routine postoperative course and be capable of recognizing problems and complications requiring the surgeon's attention.

Be sure to ask about the nurse's experience with your procedure(s).

> Being catered to in one of these posh post-op retreats can make you feel like a kid again—sort of like ice cream we all got as a reward when we had our tonsils taken out. Of course, feeling like a kid again, and especially looking like a kid (or at least like the youngest possible version of the present you), is what cosmetic surgery is all about.
>
> -Kathy Keeton, author
> *Longevity: The Science of Staying Young*

For those patients desirous of complete care outside the home, there is the "hideaway" alternative. Most large cities have specialized postoperative facilities that care for patients after cosmetic surgery. Hideaways are professionally staffed, hotel-like facilities offering appropriate meals plus transportation to the doctor's office for postoperative visits. Not to be confused with a nursing or convalescent home, the distinct purpose of a hideaway is to cater to patients recovering from cosmetic surgery. Frequently, patients who have their procedures out-of-town will opt for the hideaway, in lieu of staying in a hotel or motel. The seclusion and freedom from all responsibility, coupled with professional care and (as desired) the camaraderie of others undergoing similar procedures is, for some, an important and valued aspect of the total experience.

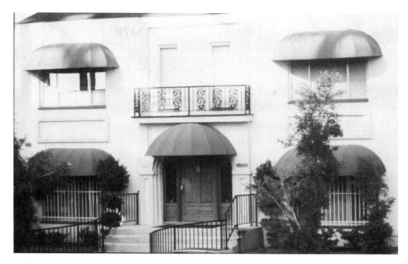

A hideaway retreat offers privacy and comfort with round-the-clock professional care and transportation to your doctor's office.

Typical Recovery Times

Recovery after cosmetic surgery is usually prompt and uncomplicated, since only superficial tissues are involved. This is in contrast to medically indicated surgery where involvement of major body cavities requires prolonged healing time. Below is a list of commonly performed cosmetic procedures and the anticipated time of recovery associated with each. Recovery time is defined as the period during which one refrains from routine social and work activities.

Nasal surgery	5 to 10 days
Ear surgery	5 to 10 days
Chin Augmentation with or without neck sculpturing	5 to 7 days
Breast Augmentation	7 to 14 days
Breast Reduction	10 to 14 days
Liposuction	5 to 14 days
Eyelid surgery	5 to 10 days
Forehead/eyebrow lift	5 to 10 days
Face and neck lift	10 to 14 days
Chemical or laser skin peel	7 to 14 days
Tummy Tuck	10 to 14 days

WHAT THE TOP COSMETIC SURGEONS DO TO HASTEN YOUR RECOVERY AND "GET YOU BACK OUT THERE"

Few people have the luxury of taking many weeks or months away from work or normal duties to recover from elective surgery. While once it *was* a matter of weeks and months before one could return to the office or feel comfortable socially, today's specialists speak of days, not weeks, and "ten to fourteen days maximum," not six to eight weeks.

How Today's Pros Do It

- Strict avoidance of aspirin, aspirin-containing compounds (you will be amazed how many products—prescription and nonprescription—have aspirin as an ingredient). See our attached list.

- Avoidance of certain homeopathic or herbal supplements that can affect blood clotting. Example: Beware the "4 Gs."*

  1. Garlic

  2. Gingko

  3. Ginseng

  4. Ginger

- Please see **Appendix D's** list of nonprescription, herbal and homeopathic drugs to be avoided.

- Use of specific medications including homeopathic medicines:

  1. **Arnica.** A homeopathic drug. Doctors prescribe it—prior to surgery and during the recovery period to reduce bruising.

  2. **Fresh Papaya and Fresh Pineapple**. Contains the enzyme papase. Helps reduce both bruising and swelling. Get to your grocery store and stock up!

---

* Edward Pribitkin, MD in *Cosmetic Surgery Times*, September 2000.

3. **Low doses of cortisone.** Safe when taken as directed for a short period of time. Extremely effective in reducing early swelling.

Postoperative Suction-Vacuum Systems

A high-tech, self-contained means to continually remove blood and tissue fluid—from under the skin—that can cause "black and blue" discoloration and tissue swelling. Typically used for one to two days after face and neck lifting, neck sculpture, forehead/eyebrow lifts, breast surgery and tummy tucks. Painless removal if done under local anesthesia.

Better Pain Control, Without The Unpleasant Side Effects

Newer medicines that stop pain in its tracks without nausea, vomiting, and that "woozy" feeling. Anesthesiologists introduce the medicines while you are asleep so that when you awaken after surgery, you are comfortable and do not require Morphine, Demerol, and other heavy narcotics.

Encourage Early Mild Exercise

Cosmetic surgeons—like their surgical brethren—found out that being bed bound for days was detrimental to a prompt recovery. Slow walking and stretching can be safely begun the day after surgery. *The longer you stay in bed, the more lethargic you become and the cycle worsens: less exercise equals more weakness, and laziness generates more bed rest.* Do not plan on running a 10K the day after your nose job, but put on your jogging shoes and at least tour the neighborhood (at sunrise or under the cover of darkness if you prefer).

Ensure Adequate Sleep

To recover quickly, you need your sleep. Often, patients sleep poorly if they have discomfort or if they are anxious, so today's cosmetic surgeons make sure their patients have the right sleep cycle by providing proper pain medicine and by insisting that they not sleep during the day. (Best way to stay awake is to get some light exercise, as mentioned above.) If you need a short-acting sleeping pill for just a night or two, that is fine. "Be awake during the day, but sleep at night."

● **Proper Diet**

To heal, you need protein. And your body needs carbohydrates and fluids to function normally. Any kind of fluids, whatever you like. When patients come in one to two days after surgery and state that they "feel weak," the first question is: "Are you eating?" Long ago, we learned that patients might not be eating because they were taking too much pain medicines that were making them nauseous. As we mentioned above, today's pain medicines are effective, and without that unpleasant side effect.

What to Expect

The timing of your first postoperative visit to the surgeon will be dependent upon the procedure(s). Face and neck lifts, tummy tucks and some breast surgery patients may be seen daily in the first few days. Less involved operations—such as nasal and eyelid procedures—typically, do not require the first visit for four to six days.

It is generally advisable to refrain from strenuous activities such as running, tennis and contact sports for seven to ten days beyond the basic recovery periods listed above.

Healing rates vary. But typically you can expect to be presentable within one to two weeks after any of these procedures. Most swelling and any bruising have usually disappeared by the seventh to tenth day. Cosmetics used for camouflage can be applied as early as three to five days following surgery. The longest period that any stitches remain in place is 14 days.

Recovery times vary: they are a function of surgical technique, type of procedure, and patient resilience. However, here are generally accepted guidelines for recovery/convalescence by procedure:

Breast Augmentation

● **Convalescence:** Home care is appropriate. No hospital- ization required.

- **Stitch Removal:** Internal absorbable stitches dissolve. If any external stitches have been placed, they are removed within seven to ten days.

- **Return to work:** Depending on the technique used, one may return to work as soon as one week after surgery—or as long as two weeks. If the breast implants are placed deep to the chest muscle, expect the longer time frame. Heavy lifting—at work or at home—is not recommended for the first three to four weeks.

- **The first week:** The dressings are removed on the first or second day after surgery. The breasts are sore; mild to moderate pain medication may be temporarily required. There may be bruising. You will require a support bra.

- **After the first week:** You should feel well enough to return to work and social activities within the second week after surgery. The swelling and soreness abates quickly. The breasts will feel firmer. The support bra may be necessary for an additional two or three weeks. If there has been any numbness, it typically disappears within a month or so. Exercise will be tolerable at two to three weeks.

Breast Lift

- **Convalescence:** Recovery at home. Mild to moderate pain is controlled with pain medicines.

- **Stitch removal:** Internal absorbable stitches dissolve. If any external stitches have been placed, they are removed within seven to ten days.

- **Return to work:** Most commonly, one week, but may be longer.

- **The first week:** Dressings may be in place for up to one week; there may be several changes to observe the healing process. Swelling and bruising begins to lessen at the end of the first week. A support bra is helpful.

- **After the first week:** Scars mature but may take up to six or even twelve months before becoming minimally visible. The complete tissue healing to yield the final result may also take many months. Smokers can expect more prolonged healing. A support bra may be necessary for several weeks.

Breast Reduction

- **Convalescence:** At home. Mild to moderate pain medication may be required.

- **Stitch removal:** Many stitches are placed—some internally—which dissolve. External stitches may be left in place up to fourteen days, depending on individual healing rates.

- **Return to work:** Two weeks is reasonable. Some patients require less while others take three weeks before returning to routine work duties. Healing and recovery time are a function of many factors including smoking, exercise, and lifestyle habits, as well as certain inherited features.

- **The first week:** Swelling, soreness, and bruising are expected. There may be some drainage from the incisions. The suction drains were inserted to reduce swelling and hasten healing. They will be removed in one to two days. A support bra is mandatory.

- **After the first week:** Scars and symmetry are the major concerns and it may be months before some temporary asymmetry settles down and the scars begin to fade. Complete scar maturation following breast reduction may take up to one year or even longer. The surgeon may recommend various medications and wound care treatments to hasten healing and minimize the visibility of the final scars. A support bra may be necessary for several weeks.

Tummy Tuck

- **Convalescence:** At home. Mild to moderate pain medication required. Because the abdominal muscles may be quite stiff and sore, you may need a bit of help getting in and out of bed for the first couple of days.

- **Stitch Removal:** External stitches are in place from five to ten or even fourteen days. Removal may be done serially—not all at once, depending on the speed of wound healing.

- **Return to work:** One to two weeks. Longer if lifting or stooping are job features.

- **The first week:** If a suction drain is used, it may be in place two days or longer. The purpose is to remove fluid that accumulates under the skin which, if not evacuated, can compromise healing and prolong swelling. Abdominal muscles are stiff and sore. You will find it difficult to flex and extend the abdomen. Bruising may be present. A corset-binder is helpful.

- **After the first week:** You may continue to use the corset-binder for several more weeks. Swelling abates and soreness disappears. If there is any bruising, it also fades rapidly. The scars will be obvious for many months and they take a year or longer to be fully mature and minimally visible. Sun protection, of course, minimizes the possibility of increased scar pigmentation during the first year or so.

Which is the Stronger Sex?

The days and weeks immediately following surgery are crucial to good results. Taking time off from work, wearing bandages, resting, avoiding the sun and strenuous activities, and saying no to alcohol and cigarettes are all important for plastic surgery patients. But these things can sometimes be difficult for men, who have been programmed by society to be stoic. Studies have shown that men often deny their pain and feel foolish about asking for help after surgery, so it is important that they have a support person available for at least a week following their operation.

– Allison Hatfield, author
"He's So Vain,"
Fort Worth, July 2001

Liposuction

- **Convalescence:** Hospital stay only if large volume of fat is removed. Otherwise at home. Mild to moderate pain medication indicated.

- **Stitch removal:** Stitch removal in five to ten days, depending on the location.

- **Return to work:** Average is one week. May be up to two weeks if large volume or multiple areas were addressed.

- **The first week:** Muscle stiffness and soreness and bruising. A compression garment is warn. Skin numbness or tingling is not uncommon.

● **After the first week:** The compression garment may be advisable for several more weeks. Bruising disappears. Sensation returns to normal. Some lumpiness is expected but typically disappears after several months. A routine exercise program can be resumed in two to three weeks.

Nasal Surgery

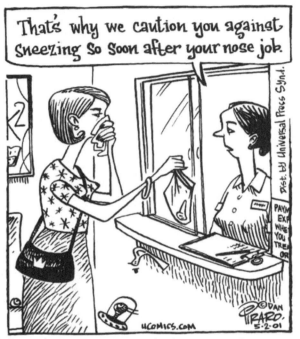

BIZARRO © 2001 by Dan Piraro. Reprinted with permission of UNIVERSAL PRESS SYNDICATE. All rights reserved.

● **Convalescence:** Home care by any responsible adult is generally adequate. You may choose to spend your first night at a hideaway retreat or hospital, but this is not necessary.

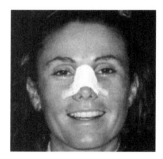

Happy — next day after surgery

● **Splint/protector and packing removal:** Since most nasal surgery is performed "internally" dissolving stitches are used. These generally do not need to be removed. The splint/protector is painlessly removed on the 4th, 5th or 6th day after surgery. Nasal packing, typically a tampon-like pad, is in place for one to five days, depening on whether or not functional surgery was also performed.

INSIDER'S INSIGHT
Aftercare - Including Nasal Pack or Stitch Removal
Need Not Be Painful

After nasal surgery, the best practices make nasal pack removal swift and painless by using old-fashioned decongestant nose drops with an added liquid anesthetic. Nothing exotic. The medicine is dribbled into the nostrils and absorbed into the nasal passages. This "shrink and numb" solution then allows the nasal pads to glide out painlessly. No torture session here. Likewise, we apply a specially compounded anesthetic ointment to eyelid and facelift incisions prior to stitch removal. Why should you have any pain at all — even during stitch removal?

For chemical or laser wrinkle removal, there are highly sophisticated and specialized anesthesia formulas available. Pain-killers are started before the patient even goes under general anesthesia, so when they wake up in the recovery room, the pain medicine is already working —keeping them comfortable. As appropriate, some patient's home care kits contain Valium. This tranquilizer, in addition to providing a relaxed, peaceful attitude the first day after surgery, also causes amnesia. As one patient remarked, "I can't remember any pain, so I guess it never happened."

Modern medicine has the answers to keep you comfortable and free from pain for the big things and even the little things. Anesthetic creams, sedatives, tranquilizers, sleeping pills, pain-killers. Superspecialists utilize all of these because they compulsively focus on every detail — before, during and after your procedure. They are driven to bring you the best total experience. The less specialized cannot do it because they are too busy pursuing a wider field of interest. Another good reason to insist on the best practices run by superspecialist surgeons.

-RK

● **Return to work:** The nose will be swollen and bruised at first, but presentable by the end of the first week. You may then return to work and normal activities providing they are not strenuous.

● **The first week:** Contact lenses can be worn one to two days after surgery. Four to six days after surgery you will be scheduled for an office visit where the outside protective shield and any remaining interior packing will be removed. If there is any bruising at this time, it should disappear within the next two to three days and can be easily concealed with makeup.

● **After the first week:** Any residual swelling will rapidly diminish. The nasal airway improves daily. Optimal breathing is generally achieved within one month.

You will probably be seen by the doctor two to three times in the first month after surgery to check healing and answer any questions. Thereafter, visits are infrequent. Postoperative photos are taken no sooner than three months after surgery.

INSIDER'S INSIGHT

In Our Practice, Tuesday Is Fun-Day

Thursday is the most popular day of the week for nasal surgery. Patients select Thursday most often because they use the weekend for recovery and can be back at work the following Wednesday or Thursday. Only four to five days off work.

A Thursday nose surgery means that the following Tuesday is the much-anticipated unveiling! Because nasal surgery requires the application of a lightweight plastic protector to avoid accidental injury, it also requires that the patient wait several days to see the result. In contrast, with breast augmentation, eyelid or facelifting, chin augmentation and other procedures, the dressings are removed within 24 hours and the result is then visible.

My staff and I share the patient's delight and wide-eyed amazement when— as the protector is quickly peeled away — the patient's new nose is revealed. Sure, it is a bit swollen and sensitive, and there is usually some mild, residual bruising. However in just five short days, the profile is straight, the bump gone. The nose is narrower; the tip more refined. The nose is already a better nose than it was less than a week earlier.

When parents, siblings, other relatives or friends are present, they share in the happiness as we hand the patient two mirrors — to see the new front view as well as their profile. We then watch that big smile evolve and the look of happy astonishment emerge.

The patient is reminded that "it only gets better" and we reinforce that by saying, "you are already looking better than you did only 120 hours (five days) ago." Copies of their "before" photos are presented as a not-too-subtle reminder of their progress.

The treatment room is a happy place; the scene of one of life's positive experiences. A smile—and occasionally even a joyful little tear. We have unwrapped a gift of lifelong satisfaction that will not wear out, needs no maintenance (except sunscreen the first three months!), and will never go out of style.

To be the creator and then the presenter of this unique gift is a very special role. In that treatment room, at that time, is where my job satisfaction is defined. This is the essence of being a physician: service to fellow man that brings happiness and comfort. My gratification compensates for the decades of late-night study, thirty-six hour training "days," and having to pass the innumerable exams necessary to be qualified and capable of delivering this most special gift.

-RK

Ear Surgery

- **Convalescence:** Home care is adequate. As with all procedures, a precise instruction/direction sheet and a "care package" of medications and supplies are provided.

- **Stitch removal:** Incisions are generally entirely behind the ear and are closed with dissolving stitches. Some stitches may take up to six weeks to dissolve.

- **Return to work:** You can return to work, school, and other normal activities three to five days after surgery. Expect the ears to be temporarily bruised, slightly swollen and sore to the touch.

- **The first week:** A helmet-type dressing is placed over the ears at surgery. It is removed the next day during a brief office visit. Small rubber drains, placed to reduce swelling and bruising, are removed from the wounds at this time. The ears are lightly redressed. Dressing can be removed at home the following day. Two days after surgery you can shower and shampoo.

- **After the first week:** It is advisable to limit strenuous exercise for three weeks, and contact sports for six weeks after surgery. To protect the newly repositioned ears, it is recommended you wear an elastic skier's headband at night for the first six weeks.

- **Over the first few months** the ears will have diminished sensation and perhaps minimal residual swelling. By three months the incisions have softened and become nearly invisible, and the ears feel "natural."

Chin Augmentation

- **Convalescence:** Convalescence at home is appropriate unless this procedure is done in conjunction with a full face and neck lift.

- **Stitch removal:** The location of your incision will be determined during consultation. It is dependent upon individual anatomy and surgeon preference. Hidden, horizontal, under-the-chin incision stitches are removed anywhere from the fourth to the sixth day after surgery. Implants can also be placed through an incision hidden inside the mouth between the lower gum and lip: stitches dissolve if the external incision is used, "steri-strips" or a "butterfly" dressing may be applied for an additional several days following stitch removal.

● **Return to work:** After one to two days it is safe to resume normal activities. If there is bruising, it can be concealed with make-up.

● **The first week:** There may be some "numbness" or slight decreased sensation about the lower lip and chin area. This will improve gradually and continue to disappear within the first several weeks. The lower lip may be stiff and swollen for a week or so.

● **After the first week:** Minimal residual swelling that will disappear completely within one month of surgery.

Neck Sculpture

● **Convalescence:** The first night can be spent either in a hideaway retreat or at home. Some surgeons place a small plastic suction tube under the skin through a tiny nick in the lower neck skin. This reduces swelling and bruising. Excess fluid collected by this drain automatically flows into a reservoir that can be managed by any responsible adult. A brief office visit is made the day after surgery. The tube is removed that day or the next.

● **Stitch removal:** Stitches are removed for the hidden, under-the-chin incision beginning on the fourth, fifth or sixth day after surgery.

● **Return to work:** You can expect to return to work and normal activities in five to seven days. Bruising can be concealed with make-up.

● **The first week:** Your neck will feel "tight" and there is slight limitation of movement for the first few days. You may experience numbness. Automobile driving is permitted after five days; this prohibition is a safety—not medical—issue since limitation of neck motion compromises your driving faculties.

- **After the first week:** Numbness about the chin and upper neck usually begins to subside. The incision may still feel lumpy, which is normal and temporary. If a chin implant has been inserted, the lower lip stiffness that may have been present initially, after surgery, begins to abate. Strenuous exercise and activities can be resumed three weeks after surgery.

- **Over the next several months** the upper neck may feel "lumpy" to the touch but is usually not visible. This condition will generally disappear in eight to twelve weeks. Within three months, the incision under the chin has matured to become fine, soft and nearly invisible. For the first six months the use of sunscreen is strongly encouraged to protect the incision and neck skin.

INSIDER'S INSIGHT

Why I Like House Calls
Occasionally, there is a good medical reason for a house call

Before I tell you about cosmetic surgery house calls, I will remind you that doctors who treat illness—family practitioners, pediatricians—did not stop visiting patients in their homes because they were lazy. They realized that apart from being able to perform a very superficial—and hence, inadequate—examination, they had little of modern science to help them diagnose and treat their patient. No lab, no x-ray.

In the heyday of house calls, there was not much technological help to be had outside the doctor's black bag. The house call was ceremonial and social, which was fine for that era of the horse and buggy.

Today, we want the best medicine rather than a dose of nostalgia and a social visit. The house is not where crucial technology lies.

Cosmetic surgery is different. We do not need CT scans, MRIs, or fancy equipment to check our patient's progress after surgery. We need what still remains the best pieces of equipment: our eyes, ears, and hands.

I have made house calls—usually on a weekend—when I was concerned about the patient's postoperative progress and if it was impractical to see them in the office. Patients appreciate house calls; some are bewildered and amazed when I say: "I'll be right over."

Now that you have revived yourself from passing out after learning that a cosmetic surgeon makes house calls, let me expand on that a bit. From my own experience, house calls have been some of the more interesting and richest aspects of my practice, and greatly appreciated by the patients. I have had a chance to visit some patients in their homes where they have shared with me personal aspects of their lives, particularly their travel experiences, or perhaps their collectibles or artwork. Such a visit is no burden—it is a learning opportunity. I have even taken one or both my daughters with me because it is a valuable life experience for them, to meet and visit interesting people in their unique habitats.

I particularly recall a house call we made one Saturday to a patient who lived in Pasadena. She was having a minor problem and it was not easy for her to get to the office that day. It is only a 25-minute drive and I promised my daughter I would take her to lunch at her favorite restaurant in Pasadena afterwards. When we came to the house, we realized we had come upon a special home with a unique, personal art collection. The woman had traveled extensively and, particularly, in Italy; she had some unusual religious artifacts. The conversation quickly turned to St. Francis of Assisi since my daughter was then doing a paper on him. Well, Lindsey never needed to open her textbook again because my patient spoon-fed her some key information and directed her to the most productive resources for research. That was over ten years ago and my daughter, when studying art history recently, happily and clearly recalled that special visit. I share this with you to remind you that medicine can be —and should be—a very personal interaction between doctor and patient. When present, that personal attachment makes medicine a very special profession.

-RK

Eyelid and Forehead/Eyebrow Lift

- **Convalescence:** The first night can be spent at a hideaway retreat or with professional home attendant. If you prefer to be at home, a precise instruction/direction sheet and "care package" of medications and supplies allows for home care by any responsible adult.

- **Stitch removal:** Upper eyelid stitches are removed between the fourth and sixth postoperative days. Lower eyelid stitches dissolve and generally do not need removal. Hidden forehead stitches may remain in place for up to ten days.

- **Return to work:** Most patients are capable of reading, writing and light activity within forty-eight hours of surgery. Normal activities can resume in five to seven days. No strenuous exercise for ten days.

- **The first week:** Any significant swelling and bruising during the first week can be concealed by wearing sunglasses. Eye make-up can be applied after stitches are removed. Eyes or brows may feel "tight"

- **After the first week:** Incisions are concealed in normal skin creases, but are slightly visible in the first four weeks following surgery. Each week their visibility is reduced until they are nearly imperceptible—about six weeks. Nightly application of a multiple vitamin ointment silicon gel is advised to promote rapid healing.

For the first several months sunscreen is strongly advised to reduce the chance of increased redness or pigmentation of the incisions as they heal.

Face and Neck Lift

- **Convalescence:** A one or two-night stay at a hideaway retreat or a professional home attendant is recommended. The complexity of a face and neck lift requires professional post-surgical observation and care. Small suction drains may be placed through tiny incisions to minimize swelling and bruising, and to speed recovery. These are best monitored and maintained by an experienced professional. Discomfort is typically minimal throughout the immediate postoperative period, but pain pills are provided if necessary. Precise instruction/direction sheets will guide you in proper care of incisions, etc.

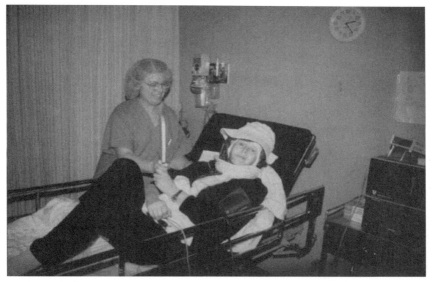

It is mid-afternoon. Our face-lift patient is about to be tranported to a recovery hideaway. Holding a hand mirror, she is already a bit curious about how she looks.

- **Two week recovery schedule:** Because of the complex nature of a full face and neck lift, recovery times are different from other procedures previously discussed.

  - **Day 1- Surgery**

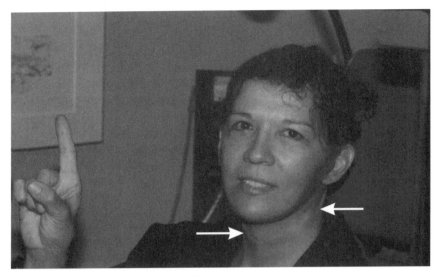

The morning after face and neck lift. Dressings have just been removed. Note minimal swelling. Arrows show location of suction tubes under the skin, which minimize swelling and bruising. The tubes are painlessly removed the following day.

- **Day 2 - Brief office visit and dressing change.** You will already appreciate a difference in your appearance.

- **Day 3- Office visit.** Dressing is changed, suction drains are removed and you return home.

- **Day 4- At home.** You may remove the dressings and shower and shampoo.

- **Day 5, 6 or 7- An office visit to remove stitches about the ears and chin.** Swelling and bruising should be minimal at this stage and you are able to be more active. Make-up can be applied. Driving privileges are restored. Walking is an excellent form of exercise at this point; however, no strenuous activities such as tennis or swimming are permitted.

- **Day 8, 9 or 10- A third office visit for further stitch removal** from the "hidden areas" (within the hairline). All bruising has typically cleared by now. You should feel quite good. You may be ready to return to work.

- **Day 14- Brief office visit.** You can fully appreciate the changes in your appearance and are ready to resume your normal activities.

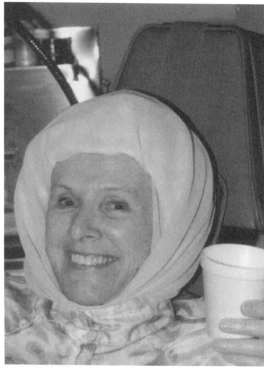

Bobbi's face and neck lift the prior day precluded her usual morning coffee. Today she is back on track.

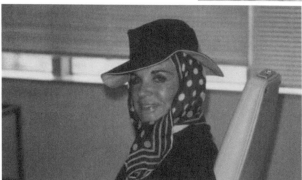

Elegant attire the morning after our lady's face and neck lift.

Chemical or Laser Skin Peel

- **Convalescence:** During the first five to seven days, your face is covered with a coating of medication. No later than the seventh day, the coating will have been washed off, revealing fresh, reddish-pink skin (akin to sunburn). By the eighth or ninth day, make-up can be applied. Appropriate skin care products, such as cleansing lotion, softening oils and sunscreens are provided by the doctor's office. Make-up techniques are also discussed.

- **The first several months:** The reddish-pink color fades naturally, and the lightening process is accelerated by medications provided. This pink color is usually gone within six to eight weeks. Any ruddy color can be concealed with cosmetics. Some people experience excessive skin dryness due to inactive oil glands, but this is easily corrected by the use of skin products provided by the doctor.

- **Going back into the sun?** Once the pink color has faded, the new skin may be slightly lighter than it was prior to the procedure and less apt to tan. Sunning is one of the most common factors of skin aging, so you will want to be vigilant about future tanning and burning. Proper sunscreens recommended by your doctor will reduce your exposure and keep your skin protected.

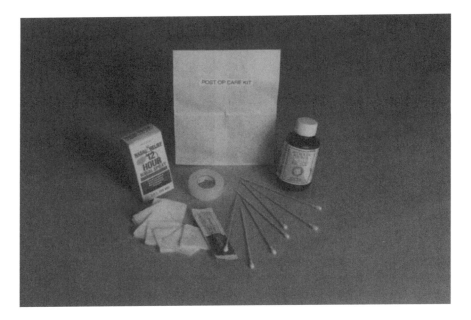

*Post-operative medication and supplies should be provided
by your surgeon.*

PATIENT COMMENTARY

I wanted to take a few moments to thank you for making my surgery as pleasing an experience as possible. From the moment I walked into your beautiful office, I knew I was in the right place. Your WONDERFUL staff took the time to walk me through all the steps of my surgery and answer every question I had. I was able to see pictures of your prior work and my projected results. I felt totally at ease with you. You made it easy to discuss exactly what I wanted and any fears I had. You explained how these changes are made and let me know exactly what my surgery would entail. As my surgery date approached, I received many calls from your office to make sure I had no further questions or concerns. The support I received from them was incredible. Your anesthesiologist even called the night before! I've never really had a major surgery, but I doubt that most patients receive this kind of thoughtful care. Everybody in the Surgicenter made sure my spirits were up and I was ready to go the morning of my surgery. I felt totally and completely unafraid. After I was home that night, I received calls from both you and your office (even the people at the surgicenter made sure I was okay). What I can tell you is that it has now been about two months since my surgery and I'm more pleased than I thought possible. I didn't want to look like another person, just improved on the old one. But the results have far exceeded anything I could have imagined.

–Melissa M, actress
California

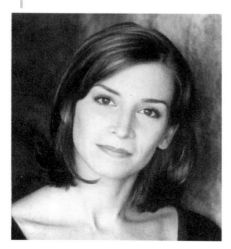

Sometimes – Even In The Most Expert Hands – Surgery Does Not Go Perfectly.

What You Need To Know. And, What To Do.

Sometimes, for reasons identifiable (or unidentifiable), complications or unsatisfactory results occur. Be mindful of the following:

- A complication should not be confused with an imperfect outcome. Before surgery, when you officially consent—in writing—to having the procedure(s) performed is when you accept possible complications; i.e., known, inherent risks such as, infection, scarring or poor healing. Not that these or other possible difficulties are likely; they are not. But in some small percentage of cases, complications or unexpected conditions do occur. Usually, they are not the fault of the surgeon, per se. Please do not blame the surgeon; he shares the anguish. Neither of you asked for this.

> **The only surgeon who has no complications is the one who never operates.**
>
> **– Aphorism well-known to all surgeons**

- Fortunately, most complications, unsatisfactory results, and disappointments can be improved upon.

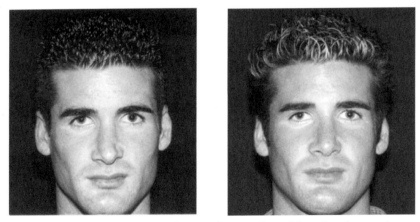

This young man had two prior nasal cosmetic and functional surgeries elsewhere. A challenging case because of the technical difficulties of operating upon twice-visited tissue.

- The competent, concerned surgeon knows what to do and will stick with you until the problem is rectified. "With you all the way." He wants you satisfied. You are his walking advertisement.

● Some imperfections or complications improve spontan-
eously, so the savvy doctor knows to allow nature some
time. This is one more way where experience counts. The
more specialized, seasoned veterans, having seen it all, have
a larger fund of experience to draw from. This helps them
better predict the course of events. These pros also tend to be
less anxious about the ultimate outcome because they know
that either nature, they themselves, or a colleague will help
correct the situation. The novice, the inexperienced
practitioner, often becomes anxious, nervous and uneasy.
This visible lack of confidence can spread to you. Your
anxiety and worry need not be compounded by your doctor.

● Your doctor should explain the problem to you, outline the
possible solutions, and suggest the best course of action.

● Often, only a minor office treatment or series of treatments
may be the solution to correct the problem.

● Your doctor may suggest a consultation with another
specialist. It may be appropriate that some or all of the
touch-up work–if necessary–be done by a specialist who has
specific knowledge and skills that should be utilized.

● There could be additional cost, particularly if another MD is
recruited. Sometimes, your health insurance is applicable.
But all financial matters should be discussed before
additional procedures are planned.

● If at any point, early or late, after a problem occurs and you
have any uneasiness, lack of confidence, or uncertainty, get
a second or even a third opinion. Your surgeon should be
willing to provide the names of specific specialists who have
the appropriate expertise. You are also free to select your
own consultant.

Consultations are valuable, if for no other reason than you may
hear from another specialist that what your surgeon is doing—or
proposes to do—makes sense. And incidentally, when you go to
another surgeon for consultation, be sure to bring copies of all your
records, including before-and-after photos. Having the complete case
history facilitates giving you an immediate, well-founded recommendation at the first visit.

The Patient is Not Responsible for an Imperfect Result

The surgeon should not make you feel responsible or ashamed for the unsatisfactory outcome or complication.

I have heard from dissatisfied patients, consulting with me, that their surgeon blamed them for the problem. One patient was told that the reason her nose was "still too wide" after rhinoplasty was that she "failed to massage it as told." How silly! Having performed over 3000 cosmetic nasal surgeries, I feel comfortable sharing this with you: In cases where the nose was not acceptably narrow in the eyes of my patient, and after the necessary time passed for swelling to reduce naturally, it was obvious to me that I had not narrowed the nasal bones and/or cartilage enough. A misjudgment on my part; not a failure of the patient.

> If there is a problem, ask the patient or family for permission to get a second opinion before they request it.
>
> – advice from Joseph Mallach, MD, one of my teachers at Northwestern Medical School, December 1966

And while massage can be helpful for the minority of cases where there is an inherent tendency for the tissues to post-operatively retain fluid, this phenomenon eventually passes. What the patient wears and bears is the sole result of the surgeon's concept, intention and execution. It is not the patient's responsibility to produce the end result. That is what you hire a cosmetic surgeon to do for you.

Such blame shifting to the innocent and now bewildered patient is not proper and suggests, to me, an immature professional. A stand-up doctor accepts responsibility for his work. When the patient is satisfied, will he not gladly accept the orchids? But, when the patient is not satisfied, he must accept the onions. He should understand that his patient is not criticizing him, only the product; he must distance himself personally from the work issue at hand.

The honorable response is to say to the patient that he does deserve an improvement from the current status and that it will be provided. No excuses, no criticism, no fiction creation, no transfer of responsibility back to the patient. The surgeon should fix it, should do the right thing.

When that proper discussion takes place—without rancor, hostility or anger—both patient and surgeon should again be relieved and comfortable with each other. A solution to a problem has been proposed and accepted. There is a plan in place. After all, the patient merely wants to know that something will be done; no one likes to be "left hanging." Particularly when the predicament was not of their creation. The top professional understands that his role does not automatically end when the last stitch of the operation is placed; it ends at the discretion of the patient—the customer, if you will—who needs to feel that everything possible has been faithfully rendered in service to him.

Do not confuse a surgeon's inappropriate criticism of patient conduct (having no bearing on the result), with a patient's willful action that compromises the outcome. The patient who smokes immediately before and after a facelift is increasing the risk of poor healing and scarring. Likewise, the nasal surgery patient who returns prematurely to contact sports and injures a fragile nose shouldn't be blaming the surgeon. You, too, have duties and the first is to heed the doctor's advice.

PATIENT COMMENTARY

Following previous unsuccessful surgery with another doctor, you reconstructed my nose on July 20, 2000. I just want to thank you so very much for my wonderful nose. I came across my before photos the other day and forgot how different I looked. You did a marvelous job! My nose looks so natural that nobody believes me that I had a nose job. But when they see my before photos, they are amazed at what a great and subtle job you did! Once again, thank you for my cute nose that is now two years and seven months old!

– e-mail received from Melissa S. on March 20, 2002
California

"Oh, doctor," said the young lady, "will the scar show?"
"That, madam," said the doctor, "is entirely up to you."
-Jacob M. Braude
Braude's Treasury of Wit and Humor

Thirty-one percent of women would consider plastic surgery either now or in the future.
– American Society for Aesthetic Plastic Surgery as quoted in
Allure Magazine

11

ERASING MENTAL BLOCKS

Secret: **There is a responsible answer or solution for every concern, worry and reservation.**

PATIENT COMMENTARY

I can now breathe much better through my nose and I'm very happy with the way it looks. My nose looks so natural that no one has been able to notice...Friends and family are amazed at how natural my nose looks. Even my mother has mentioned how my nose complements the rest of my facial features.

-Christian, traffic specialist
Florida

PATIENT COMMENTARY

My final decision to have surgery came when I received a letter from my 81-year-old aunt who just had cataract surgery. She said, "If there's anything that you need to change, don't wait as long as I did. Do it as soon as possible."

-Susan
California

PATIENT COMMENTARY

I had some hesitation myself. But I had one big advantage. I had listened carefully to our patients relating their experiences. Over and over, I heard the following phrase: "You know, this wasn't such a big deal. I don't know why I worried about it. Why did I wait so long?" We all magnify our worries and concerns out of proportion; most of the things we worry about in life never happen. Worry is the misuse of imagination. Still, we all worry about 'going to sleep,' particularly for an elective procedure. But again, what I knew is that I was safer in a licensed surgery center with a doctor-anesthesiologist at my side than I am during my freeway commute. Those statistics are absolute! Further, Dr. Kotler will not operate unless the patient "passes" the required pre-operative physical and lab tests. No one should have elective surgery unless he or she is medically fit. So if you are healthy for this kind of surgery, your risk is nearly zero.

-Karel Rall
Patient Counselor
Cosmetic Surgery Specialists
Medical Group of Beverly Hills

If cosmetic surgery is as positive and satisfying as it sounds, why isn't everyone having it done?

Some people cannot have the surgery they desire—under any circumstances—because of a dangerous medical condition. They will be informed of this during the requisite physical prior to any surgery being scheduled.

Other people have been blessed with satisfactory "architecture" and practice a healthy lifestyle: staying trim, avoiding nicotine, exercising regularly, eating a well balanced diet, drinking moderately, and protecting their skin from excessive sun. These people may not need anything done. In either case, the reputable practitioner tells the patient they are not a good candidate for cosmetic surgery, and explains why.

There then remains a third group: healthy, but not happy with their inherited features or appearing older than they prefer. They long for a better appearance but are so ambivalent, they can't make the commitment. In our practice survey patients were asked, "How long have you been considering cosmetic surgery?" The range of answers was three months to ten years! The median time period was three years. Events, functions, vacations, and assorted obligations come first. Unlike a broken leg or gallbladder attack, the elective nature of cosmetic surgery makes it easy to put off. Often, however, the ambivalence and hesitation stem from mistaken notions and misformation, about cosmetic surgery.

Interestingly, we find surprising consistency among prospective patients when asked to identify reasons that kept them from having surgery. Here are the seven most frequently stated concerns, hesitations and blocks.

1. "I'm afraid. The idea of having any surgery and anesthesia scares me."

2. "What will I look like? Will the results be natural?"

3. "How long before I can return to social activities, work or exercise?"

4. "Will it be painful?"

5. "What will my family, friends or coworkers think about this?"

6. "Can I afford what I want?"

7. "Which doctor is best qualified for my particular case?"

All these questions pose legitimate and proper concerns. The responses may provide you with the information and reassurance you need to remove your mental blocks:

1. "I'm afraid. The idea of having any surgery and anesthesia scares me"

All cosmetic surgery procedures are anatomically superficial. They involve only the skin and the tissues just below the skin. These procedures are not comparable in any way to major abdominal surgery, open-heart surgery, or brain surgery. Regardless of the procedure, you are an outpatient and will leave the surgery center one to two hours after the operation. Should you be having nose, chin, eyelid surgery or breast augmentation early in the morning, you can expect to be home by lunch!

PATIENT COMMENTARY

> *The nasal surgery itself was a piece of cake! I didn't even use the pain pills you gave me! It was one of the easiest and greatest decisions I have ever made.*
>
> *-Karen, beautician*
> *California*

2. "What will I look like? Will the results be natural?"

Unnatural, overdone, plastic-looking cosmetic surgery does not come from "bad luck." It is the result of poor surgeon selection. Why would anyone not want to look natural? Everyone recognizes those celebrities who have been over-tightened, over-pulled and over-sculpted. They simply do not look natural. The best practices assure the patients that their results will be as natural as those shown in their "before and after" album. That's why I'm so keen on your examining the real-life or photographic evidence of a doctor's work.

Caveat emptor! Buyer beware!

INSIDER'S INSIGHT

A Tale of a Dissatisfied Patient - How You Can Avoid a Similar Error of Judgment

Prospective Patient at Consultation:

Several months ago, my friend had a facelift and I must say she does not look good. I'm shocked. First, it is obvious something's been done to her face because it does not look natural. It's like her face is always smiling. She has a constant grin — like The Joker in Batman. And when she smiles or speaks, she gets these strange, horizontal grooves in her face. It looks terrible. If this is what cosmetic surgery does, it's not for me. But I need to ask you: What did my friend do wrong? How do I know it won't happen to me?

I don't blame you for being concerned. Your friend's appearance may well be due to having had a type of face lift that, if *overdone,* causes permanent distortion of the facial features because it involves repositioning many of the muscles and their attachments to the underlying bones. Or, the 'lifting' of the skin—involving a backward pull—may have been overdone, although, typically, if that is the cause, time should improve the appearance.

Your friend did not cause these deformities—the surgeon did. It seems his judgment was poor because no one wants an overdrawn, distorted and unnatural result. An experienced cosmetic surgeon knows this and avoids the problem by not performing a procedure that can possibly create such an outcome. These poor results don't 'just happen' with a qualified, experienced cosmetic surgeon.

If your friend is unhappy, she might look to her decision-making process when she selected the doctor. Did she see other patients whose facelifts were done by the doctor she chose? Did she see the surgeon's before-and-after photo collection? Did the doctor show her—using a computer imaging program—what he intended to accomplish? And did she see examples of patients' actual results   compared with the computer predictions?

The doctor should have a standard or routine technique he uses for his facelifts. Most likely, then, all his patients will look unappealing to a prospective patient. That is why it is so important to see multiple examples—either "live," or in "before and after" photos—of the doctor's results. If you don't like the results you are seeing, go elsewhere.

-RK

Modern cosmetic surgery is capable of delivering far better than this lady's friend received. You should not have to worry about wearing the equivalent of a neon sign on your face that proclaims: "Bad Cosmetic Surgery." If every patient had cosmetic surgery by the appropriate superspecialist who performs cosmetic surgery only, the percentage of dissatisfied patients would be very, very low.

3. "How long before I can return to social activities, work or exercise?"

If you have nose, chin or eyelid surgery, you can be back to work and/or be "seen in public" within one week. Figure ten days for facelifts, wrinkle removal or combination procedures. Strenuous exercise can be done in ten to fourteen days, but walking is encouraged three to four days after any procedure. Not bad.

PATIENT COMMENTARY

Having my nose done is probably one of the best decisions I've ever made. If only I could have done it sooner!! I was extremely amazed at the short recovery and how much of an impact this surgery has made on my life.

-Jerre, sports trainer
California

PATIENT COMMENTARY

It is just eight days since my neck surgery and, although there is a little bruising, it looks superb and I feel great. Thanks again.

-Bobbie, businesswoman
California

P.S. When do I start to feel pain?

4. "Will it be painful?"

INSIDER'S INSIGHT

"Doctor, one of the worries that has kept me from this consultation for years is having heard the horror stories about pack removal after nasal surgery."

The patient is referring to reports of pain when the internal nasal packs — long gauze strips or finger-like cotton pads — are removed one or several days after surgery. Likewise, when I suggest to patients with wrinkles, that chemical rejuvenation would be an appropriate solution, I hear, "Oh, I heard it hurts too much", or, "My friend had one and did nothing but complain about the pain. I'd rather live with the wrinkles."

I am irked by the "bad press" our specialty gets because many of us do it right every day. In the 21st century there is no excuse for patients to suffer in surgery or during recovery. Prospective patients need to hear how the pros do it. The negative stories come from amateur — not superspecialist — offices. There is time, and there are medicines, to do it properly — painlessly.

-RK

PATIENT COMMENTARY

> *I have no recollection of pain at all; not during the surgery, not after surgery. I did not take any pain pills. The only thing that reminded me about the surgery was my swollen nose. But the swelling went away soon.*
>
> *-Natalia, artist*
> *California*

In this day and age, if a doctor cannot control pain, he should retire. Safe, effective pain medications are widely available. They won't create addiction; they're only used for a short time. You should be provided, as part of your service, a medium strength pain medicine such as Tylenol© with codeine or Vicodin©. The majority of patients require nothing stronger. If these are not effective or cause side effects, there are many substitutes. No physician should let you suffer! Keep your doctor apprised of your status, and if you're experiencing pain, don't hesitate to call the office. The best practices are available 24 hours a day to insure your comfort. Prior to surgery, be sure you have all the phone numbers to reach the surgeon or one of his staff at any time.

5. "What will my family, friends, or co-workers think about this?"

Is it really important what others think? It's your face or body. What is important is what you think. Don't put it out for a vote. *If you want it, "just do it!"*

PATIENT COMMENTARY

> *I want to thank you for the new me. I look so much younger, I just can't believe it. My skin is new and wrinkle-free! It feels great to look as young as my daughters again! I know that coming to you for my chemical peel was one of the best things I've ever done for myself. Sam was skeptical before I had the peel; now he takes all the credit for it! He says he might even keep me around a few more years. Thanks again for the new skin! I love it! Sincerely,*
>
> *-Glenda, insurance broker*
> *Tennessee*

6. "Can I afford what I want?"

The popularity of cosmetic surgery is testimony to its value and affordability. It is no longer an exclusive indulgence of the rich and famous. Interest in cosmetic surgery spans into most socioeconomic levels of American society. Don't let money alone stand between you and your appearance. Think of it as an investment in your future.

INSIDER'S INSIGHT
The Daily Cost of a Teenager's Nose Job

When a teen has a nose job at age 17, she can expect to live another 64 years to age 81. So, let's do some math and see what it costs, per day—to own a great nose. Take the total cost of the cosmetic nasal surgery (including surgeon's fees, outpatient surgery center charges, anesthesiologist fees), divide it by the remaining life span of the teen, and divide by 365 days in a year. That gives you the cost per day.

Sample Calculation:

Lindsey, a 17 year-old high school student wants to have her nose done. She needs to convince her parents to fund it. Finally finding a practical use for math she makes the following calculation:

- Her predicted life span=81 years.
- Subtract current age of 17 from 81=64. She can expect 64 years to enjoy her new nose.
- Assume: total cost of the surgery is $6000.
- Divide $6000 by 64 years=$94 per year!
- Divide $94/year by 365 days/year=26 cents per day! Less than a local telephone call!

-RK

Earlier, I revealed strategies to soften the expense without compromising quality. Here are more ideas to make surgery available to you with less financial sacrifice.

"Stand by" fees

For patients who have a flexible work schedule and can be available with seven to ten days notice, some practices offer significant cost savings. A surgeon's operating schedule is most efficient when all the spaces are filled. Airlines offer discounted seats—surgeons can do the same. Be sure to ask about "stand by" rates.

...people have been haggling for years over the cost of things insurance doesn't usually pay for, such as plastic surgery...

Wall Street Journal,
February 8, 2002

"Friends and family" group discounts

This popular concept is great for groups. When sisters, cousins, or friends consult together and have their procedures on the same or successive days, each member of the group saves money. First, it costs the practice no more to consult with four people than it does with one. Next, pre- and post-operative care is very efficient and a cost-saver when several people have the procedures done in tandem. The practice's savings are passed along to you.

"Layaway" plans

Layaway plans are a great way to save towards a purchase and earn a bonus at the same time. Here's how it works. Each month for twelve months, you send in a pre-determined payment. When you have reached the eleventh month, the practice will reward you with a discount or bonus towards your final payment. You are then paid up and ready for your cosmetic surgery of choice!

Financing plans

National consumer credit companies offer financing for cosmetic and dental surgery as well as other elective professional services. Most practices have a relationship with these companies and can provide you with application forms either online or by fax. Often, you can expect an answer within hours.

Credit Cards

Credit cards are perhaps the most practical and common means of financing purchases. Some practices accept major credit cards. Patients enjoy getting "free miles" along with their new face and body.

Company Credit Unions

If you work for an employer with a credit union, borrowing there may be your best deal. Credit union interest rates tend to be lower than credit cards.

PATIENT COMMENTARY

It's the first time in my life I purchased something and got exactly what I wanted and far more than I expected.

-Mishel,* controller, production company
California

* See Mishel's photo on page 109.

7. Which doctor is best qualified for my particular case?"

You need to be very comfortable with your decision: Follow the dictates of this book and you will be. There is no more critical factor than selecting the most experienced and narrowly specialized surgeon possible. Surgical outcomes are directly related to the experience, skill and degree of specialization of the practitioner. The surgeon who does not focus on the particular procedure you are considering should be excluded from consideration. And, right there, don't be reluctant to ask for a referral to a colleague who does specialize in that procedure. A conscientious and competent practitioner will admit he is not comfortable with your case. He will then make a recommendation that you consult with one or more of his colleagues whose work is familiar to the doctor.

Keep in mind, there is seldom "good luck" or "bad luck" in cosmetic surgery. You can do your homework, or roll the dice. Your choice.

> **The definition of a professional is one who puts the interest of the client (patient) ahead of his own.**
>
> **-Louis Brandeis**
> **U.S. Supreme Court Justice**

APPENDIX A

Accessory Techniques and Products for Aging Skin

Products That "Fill" or Affect Grooves, Deep Wrinkles and Some Scars

Some unsatisfactory aspects of facial structure can be superficially improved by what we cosmetic surgeons call "soft tissue augmentation." That is medicalese for "plumpers and fillers" placed under the skin by doctors to aid in rejuvenation.

> The best product in the world is only as good as the person using it. Only time will tell which products provide the best results and the fewest drawbacks.
>
> **-Arnold Klein, MD**

Typically, these are minor office procedures. Here is the short list of some of the more popular products.

Collagen Injections—Collagen is a naturally occurring substance within the skin and is a principle contributor to the skin's strength and smoothness. It can be used to improve facial lines, creases, grooves and some scars. Collagen injections are used as "fillers." It also works for "indentations" such as the deep crease between the cheeks and lip.

> The American Society of Plastic Surgeons reports use of collagen injections climbed by 28% between 1992 and 1999.

The substance is injected into and underneath the skin and takes effect immediately. Because it is derived from animal tissue that is not living, the body digests and eliminates it. Therefore, it is necessary for your doctor to perform "refills" every three or four months. Collagen has been available for over twenty years and has proven itself to be safe, practical and effective. However, each patient should be tested for sensitivity or allergy to this nonhuman substance. This is done by a simple skin test, similar to a tuberculosis skin test. The results will demonstrate whether there is sensitivity to the product or not. Inamed Aesthetics markets the most popular collagen products: Zyplast® and Zyderm®.

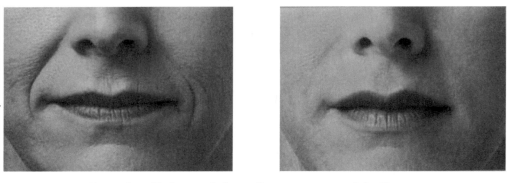

Photos courtesy of Inamed Aesthetics

Examples of before and after collagen treatment of the lips.

Fat Injections—Fat injection techniques are still in a state of evolution. Theoretically, fat would be an ideal substance to fill deep creases and grooves in the face and replace the missing fat, which shrinks in the natural course of aging. However, the perfect solution for using fat transplantation has been somewhat elusive. The fat is harvested using a liposuction-type technique from hidden areas such as the lower abdomen or buttocks. It is then injected into the facial areas that need it. The challenge of this procedure has been to perfecting the technique to maximize transplanted fat survival, minimize absorption, and eliminate lumpiness and irregular ties.

Isolagen®—This is a preparation used to act as a "filler" in areas where creases, grooves and lines are becoming problematic. The injection is derived from processed cells taken from one's own skin. Though the process promises to be effective, it has not yet gained major popularity among cosmetic surgeons and dermatologists. It should be noted that at the time of this writing, it has been placed on hold by the FDA.

Alloderm®—A tissue graft of human skin from which the living cells have been removed. It comes in sheets and is incorporated into the tissues over a period of time. Depending on the area being treated, the Alloderm graft can be rolled or folded to suit the particular need. Cymetra® is the refined version of Alloderm®.

> **Beauty is only skin deep, but the impression it makes is not.**
>
> **-Evan Esar**
> *20,000 Quips & Quotes*

> The world of filler substances has undergone a small revolution over the last several years and many more substances are now available for soft tissue augmentation. As a physician, one has one's own idea of what would make the ideal filler substance. Nothing as of yet fulfills all expectations, but there are many more substances that can be very useful. . .One would prefer to have the substance that has little risk of allergy reaction. One would like it to be relatively long lasting, but not necessarily permanent, so that should a patient have an untoward effect or dislike the implant, he or she can be assured that it is not to be a permanent situation. One would like it to be painless for the patient and quite easy to use for the physician. . . One would like it to be inexpensive and have reproducible results. One would like it to have minimal side effects such as bruising, irritation, infection, migration, or tissue reaction and loss. In the United States, one would prefer that the material be approved by the Food and Drug Administration (FDA). *There is no substance at this time that can fill all of these requirements.*
>
> -Robin Ashinoff, MD
> "Overview: Soft Tissue Augmentation,"
> in *Clinics in Plastic Surgery*, October 2000

GoreTex®— Most people recognize GoreTex® as a fabric-like material used for many commercial purposes, including skiwear. In cosmetic surgery, GoreTex® cloth is tunneled underneath the skin and acts as a "filler." Over a period of time, natural tissue migrates around the material and infiltrates to stabilize it. Insertion requires small imperceptible incisions. In a small percentage of patients, the man-made material will not be tolerated and must be removed.

SoftForm®—This is a hollow tube of synthetic material that is inserted through small hidden incisions about the face and is also used to fill grooves and depressions. Natural tissue grows within the hollow of the tube helping to stabilize it. It must be placed deep enough under the skin so as not to be visible and yet not so deep as to be ineffective.

Hyaluronic Acid—Hyaluronan is a naturally occurring substance in our bodies. As we get older, hyaluronan decreases and the skin becomes less taut and more dry. Hyaluronic acid increases the level of hyaluronan when injected into the skin. Since there is no species specificity, no skin testing is necessary, although reactions have been reported with both Restylane® and Hylaform® gel, the two most frequently used hyaluronic acid products.

Silicone—Medical-grade silicone is a clear, oil-like liquid that has been successfully used to fill grooves, depressions and raised scars on the face for decades. Because of the silicone breast implant controversy, many practitioners abandoned it. However, silicone in experienced hands can be safe and effective. Recently, **Silicone 1000** (Alcon Corporation) was approved for certain medical uses. Cosmetic surgeons use it for many indications, including select wrinkles and certain acne scars.

> The Baby Boomer population is demanding products and procedures to treat skin problems associated with aging. The emphasis on how we can help our skin will follow the trend toward reversing aging and slowing down future damage.
>
> -Susan E. Downey, MD, USC Associate Professor of Clinical Surgery *USC Health,* 2001

"Lite" Chemical Peeling Agents

Alpha-hydroxy Acids—These mild peeling agents act as a deep exfoliant removing the dead cells from the skin surface and accelerating the maturation of the remaining cells. The aim is to make the skin smoother to the touch and more lustrous in appearance. The most commonly used alpha-hydroxy acids are lactic acid, glycolic acid and citric acid. Alpha-hydroxy acids (in concentrations of less than 10 percent) are used in cosmetic preparations; in concentrations of 10-to 70 percent, as skin peeling agents. Some of the alpha-hydroxy acids commonly recognized are: ascorbic acid, citric acid, glycolic acid, lactic acid, malic acid and tartaric acid. These acids are naturally occurring in citrus fruits, milk, tomatoes, apples, mangoes, grapes and sugar cane.

In antiquity, women bathed themselves in sour milk in the hope of softening and smoothing the skin. Perhaps they understood intuitively that sour milk contains lactic acid, now used for the same purpose.

Beta-hydroxy Acids—These contain salicylic acids which have affects similar to alpha-hydroxy acids. Beta-hydroxy acid-containing products include Oil of Olay's Age Defying Series and the Medicis Pharmaceutical's Beta-Lift® skin peel.

Medium Strength Chemical Peels

The most common medium strength agent is trichloroacetic acid ("TCA"). Typically used in concentrations between 20 percent and 50 percent, TCA, a strong acid, destroys the epidermis (the outer layer of skin) and penetrates into the dermis (deeper skin). As a result, it stimulates the formation of new, fresh skin that is richer in collagen and elastic fibers, and is more taut with fewer wrinkles. Trichloroacetic acid has been used by experienced practitioners for many years. Because of the strength of this chemical and the possibility of complications, TCA skin peels should be performed only by experienced dermatologists and cosmetic surgeons. Anesthesia may be required for patient comfort and safety. This process of skin rejuvenation may take five to seven days of "down time" after which the skin is red. Cosmetics are required until the red color fades. When red, the skin is extremely sensitive to the effects of the sun and, therefore, a comprehensive skin program emphasizing sun protection is mandatory.

The "Heavy Hitters"

Laser Peels

Laser resurfacing utilizes modern technology to treat sun-damaged and aging skin. The invisible, high-energy light beam destroys the outer layer of skin by boiling the water within the skin cells. This causes the formation of new, young, fresh and smooth skin. There is a broad variety of laser technology.

> **Wrinkles should merely indicate where smiles have been.**
>
> -Mark Twain

The most commonly used lasers are carbon dioxide (CO_2) lasers for aggressive skin resurfacing of the entire face and Erbium: YAG lasers. Carbon dioxide lasers affect the deeper portions of the skin. The heat causes new collagen to form. Erbium lasers vaporize superficial portions of the skin. Therefore, it is hoped that a combination of both (Erbium:YAG and CO_2) may prove to be the most effective.

The Nd:YAG (Neodynium) laser—is becoming popular for superficial wrinkles. It penetrates below the outer layer of skin stimulating fresh collagen without causing a destruction of the outer most layers. This translates into a shorter healing time. But this procedure, because it is less intense, requires maintenance treatments and has not lasted as long other laser treatments. This is considered a "nonablative" laser technique: it does not peel or damage the outer layer of skin. The target is the sun-damaged collagen and elastic fibers in the upper dermis just beneath the outer epidermis layer. Further research is in progress.

Coblation. Appropriate only for mild to moderate skin wrinkling. This is a variant of laser technology that improves the appearance of the skin by heating the below-the-surface collagen causing it to reform into tighter bands. The purported advantage – compared to established resurfacing by CO2 and YAG laser and chemical peels – is more rapid healing translating to shorter recovery time. Because there is less damage to the skin surface. Cool Touch, Visage, N-Lite, Smooth Beam, and Aramis are currently some of the systems being investigated and evaluated.

> "Outward appearance can indeed affect inner feelings and self-esteem," says Dr. Eugenie Brunner, an eminent plastic surgeon in Princeton, New Jersey. "It can't make you look like someone else or guarantee job success or make people like you. What it can do is improve the harmony and balance of your facial features, reverse some of the signs of aging, and help you look your best."
>
> from *Don't Count the Candles*
> by Joan Rivers

Deep Phenol Peels

Phenol peels, the so-called "heavyweight champions" of skin rejuvenation, have a long and successful history. They have been performed in the U.S. as a mainstream procedure since the early 1960s.

Phenol is an acid-like chemical that, when mixed with other agents, becomes a potent prescription that resurfaces the skin by removing wrinkles, crow's feet, age spots and other superficial skin imperfections. Experienced practitioners regard phenol formulations as the standard against which all other skin resurfacing procedures must be measured.

Because of its ability to penetrate to the deeper layers, there will be some permanent lightening of the skin in everyone except those with the fairest complexions. This categorically rules out patients of color, as well as those who don't want to wear makeup to camouflage the color-different zone of transition between the treated face and untreated neck. Because of the same color issue, most men are excluded unless they are comfortable wearing bronzing solutions for camouflage or wear a beard.

You can see photographic examples and further description of the deep phenol peel in **Chapter 6,** which has been described by patients as "astounding," "amazing," and "unbelievable." I have performed the procedure for over 30 years and I am still in awe each time the patient returns for the one-week visit. By then the process of

Six Signs of Aging Skin:

- **Fine lines and wrinkles**
- **Blotches and age spots**
- **Poor skin texture**
- **Poor skin tone**
- **Increased dryness**
- **Visible pores**

skin rejuvenation and healing is complete and the result is "almost magical.*"

Because phenol application is painful, the procedure should be performed under surgical conditions, with general anesthesia administered by a nurse anesthetist or physician anesthesiologist. Within eight to twelve hours of application, the phenol anesthetizes the nerve endings and there is little pain. However, immediately following the procedure, strong pain medicine must be available to the patient. Typically, the patient has dressings applied to the skin allowing the phenol solution to penetrate into the most wrinkled and crevice-like areas. These are removed under a short intravenous sedation forty-eight hours after treatment. For the next five days, the process of "shedding" the aged skin layer takes place. By day six or seven, resurfacing is complete and the new, fresh, smooth, wrinkle-free skin is apparent.

Botulinum Toxin

Botox Cosmetic® and Myobloc™. Treatment of hyperfunctional lines with botulinum toxin occupies a unique and welcome role in facial rejuvenation. Neither Botox Cosmetic® nor Myobloc™ "fills in " nor "puffs out" grooves and creases; they are not filling materials. These muscle weakeners are very effective on the forehead and between the eyebrows, the site of strong, repeated muscle contraction. The drugs paralyzing effect temporarily blocks nerve transmission, thereby lessening muscle tension and relaxing the tissues.

Botox Cosmetic® and Myobloc™ are office treatments. The result takes three to five days to manifest and the benefits last from three to six months. Some surgeons are experimenting with Botox® Cosmetic to reduce prominence of the vertical muscle cords of the neck (platysma bands).

As Botox Grows in Popularity—So Do The Jokes

In April 2002 Allergen, the manufacturer of Botox Cosmetic®, announced that the FDA (Food and Drug Administration) had

---

* Neil Baum, MD

approved the use of Botox® Cosmetic for the treatment of glabeller lines (brow furrows).

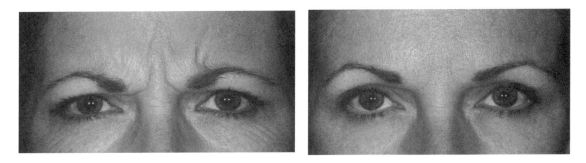

Left, patient using forehead muscles before botox injection, Right, same expression after Botox injection. (Photos courtesy of American Academy of Dermatology and Drs. Robert and Margaret Weiss.)

Here are some insightful commentaries and quotes from Maureen Dowd's article on the subject in the *New York Times,* February 10, 2002:

● *Anna Quidlen notes that 'it is now rare in certain social enclaves to see a woman over the age of 35 with the ability to look angry.'*

● *In the immortal words of Patricia Wexler, a New York dermatologist who caters to uncrinkled celebrities: 'A scowl is a totally unnecessary expression.'*

● *Actresses are caught in a cosmetic Catch-22. they must look young to get juicy roles, so they do Botox, which makes it impossible to play juicy roles.*

● *We may be at war with terrorists, but the cover of the new People magazine is a post-eye-job, creaseless Greta Van Susteren, who proclaims that with her plastic surgery, 'I've made it safe for other people.'*

● *As one journalist drolly notes, 'Tim Russert is the last person standing in network news who can definitely still scowl.'*

> **If Botox can erase all those years… there's no reason not to let it. From a medical standpoint, experts says there's little harm involved. "Botox is win-win because there is little discomfort and it is extremely low risk," says Malcolm Paul, MD, president of the American Society for Aesthetic Plastic Surgery.**
>
> **-"Botox Babies,"**
> *Mademoiselle Magazine*

● *New York doctors are already envisioning princess-to-frog (or dog) scenarios in which men marry smooth-faced women and, four months and no Botox injections later, wake up next to a Shar-Pei.*

Anti-Aging Creams — Dreams Fulfilled

Age I do abohor thee; youth, I do adore thee.
                    -William Shakespeare

> **Age is an issue of mind over matter. If you don't mind, it doesn't matter.**
>
> **-Mark Twain**

Tretinoin or retinoic acid— This prescription product is available in liquid, cream or gel form, and in varying concentrations. Originally, it was used as an acne treatment; the stronger concentrations are effective in improving skin quality to minimize fine wrinkles, irregular pigmentation and skin roughness. This Vitamin A derivative carries considerable potency and the possibility of side effects. Retinoic acid can be combined with other prescription medications to become even more effective, particularly as a bleaching agent. Retinoic acid causes dryness and scaling. Hence, it must always be combined with a comprehensive skin care program including moisturizers and sunscreens, particularly since retinoic acid renders the skin more sensitive to the effects of sun. Products include Retin-A®, Renova® and Avita®.

Retinol—Retinol, is a pure form of Vitamin A that, it is believed, undergoes conversion to tretinoin (retinoic acid) in the skin. Because the conversion yields a less-concentrated version of tretinoin, it appears to be less irritating but is also probably less effective. Retinol products include Neutrogena Healthy Skin® anti-wrinkle cream and Roc Retinol Active Pure ™.

Poly-hydroxy Acids—Poly-hydroxy acids, which consist of large alpha-hydroxy acid molecules, were designed to slow down penetration thereby causing less redness and irritation. Dermatologists have found no significant differences between the effects of alpha-hydroxy and poly-hydroxy acids. Poly-hydroxy acid products include the Neostrata NeoCeuticals® line.

Topical estrogen—When applied directly onto the skin, estrogen, the female hormone, may reverse signs of aging in postmenopausal women. Additional research is needed to confirm this hormone's benefit.

Elastica®—Shows promise for reviving elastin, a major structural skin component (the other is collagen). This cream contains an extract from cow's ligaments.

Kinerase®—This is an over-the-counter product used topically to improve the appearance and smoothness of skin. The product is chemically unique in that it is not a drug or an exfoliant. It appears to act by delaying the biochemical processes which contribute to skin aging. The side effects are minimal. Because this is a newer product, more extensive evaluation is necessary to fully understand its function and promise.

AFAs® or amino fruit acids—These are not fruit acids, such as glycolic or lactic acid or the other alpha-hydroxy acids. Through a biochemical process, these substances become effective antioxidants. In a gel vehicle, they are usually nonirritating and nonallergic. The aim of this product is to increase moisture retention within the skin aswell as to improve the tone and texture. It affects the outer layer of skin. An increased benefit may be a decreased sensitivity to sunlight and, hence, less chance for pigmentary changes.

Smoking: Your Skin's Mortal Enemy
Is Smoking Very Bad or Just Bad?

Studies have found that smoker's skin does have dramatically damaged elastic fibers, even on areas that have never seen the light of day.

BUT

Smokers seem to wrinkle only in sun-exposed areas and if smoking were integral to sagging, cigarette addicts would wrinkle all over, points out Steven Feldman, MD, Associate Professor of Dermatology and Pathology at Wake Forrest University School of Medicine.

-from Tri. H. Nguyen, MD,
Assistant Professor of Dermatology

Topical Vitamins – The Newest Frontier

Vitamin C (ascorbic acid)—Recently, topical forms of this well-known vitamin have been incorporated into chemicals that rejuvenate the skin. The method of action is not certain. It may be that Vitamin C may help reduce the ultraviolet light-induced oxygen-free radicals, which contribute to skin aging. In this manner, it may serve to offer skin protection from ultraviolet rays just as sunscreens do. Cellex-C® is the most common commercial preparation.

Vitamin E— The topical form of Vitamin E is alpha-tocopherol. It functions as an antioxidant and therefore retards the aging of the surface skin.

The Latest Office Skin Care Treatment Procedures

Microdermabrasion. 21 manufacturers marketing 54 different machines, including Delphia, Crystal Peel, Cellabrasion, Europeel, Propeel, Diamond Peel, Smart Peel and Dermaglide. This is a high-tech, delicate, "sandblasting" of the skin to soften and remove very superficial blemishes. It is a mechanical skin exfoliation, a buffing, using a stream of tiny crystals. It is performed in salons and some dermatology offices. The potency of this product matches that of the lightest chemical peels. Plan on several treatment sessions.

Intense Pulse Light. Similar to a laser beam. Used to erase pigment and to decrease redness of certain medical skin conditions such as rosacea or after chemical or laser peeling. Effective against tiny facial blood vessels. Expect four or more treatments. Some of the more common systems available are the Fotofacial™, Prolite, Vasculight™ and Quantum SR.

Three Simple Things You Can Do To Save Your Skin

1. *Don't smoke.* Cigarette smoke, with its nicotine and carbon dioxide (among other noxious elements), causes the skin's blood vessels to constrict and narrow, and thus chokes off the flow of oxygen and other nutrients to the skin. With every cigarette, the skin dies a little bit.

2. *Protect your skin from the sun.* Use sunscreens or sunblocks if your skin is particularly sensitive. If you live in sun-intensive climates of Southern Texas, Florida, and California, your skin will be assaulted year-round. If you live in Duluth, Minnesota, don't worry.

3. *Pick the right parents.* If your parents have smooth, unwrinkled skin as seniors, it augurs well for you.

SMOKING and WRINKLES

Cosmetic surgeon Robert Kotler, MD, discovered smokers were three times more likely to develop deep wrinkles. He found that a third of those who smoked were severely wrinkled, but only 12 percent of non-smokers were.

'Smoking causes blood vessels in the skin to constrict, depriving tissue of nutrition,' Dr. Kotler explains. 'That means less blood flow to the largest organ in the body, the skin. That's why smokers' skin looks older, more wrinkled and is of poorer quality.'

-from "Anatomy of a Wrinkle,"
by Paddy Calistro, in *For Women First*

Aging Skin And Skin Care Questionnaire
True Or False?

1.   Surgical facelifts remove wrinkles.

2.   Too much sun is bad for the skin.

3.   Using creams and oils will remove wrinkles.

4.   Facial exercises may help retard the aging process.

5.   Good skin is partially dependent on heredity.

6.   Excess face washing with soap may be harmful to the skin.

7.   Where you live may be a factor in how quickly your skin ages.

8.   Cigarette smoking may make skin age prematurely.

9.   Dark skin resists wrinkling.

10. X-ray treatment to the skin may cause premature wrinkling.

11. Baby oil is worthless as a sunscreen agent.

12. Certain prescription or nonprescription items can affect your skin's reaction to the sun.

13. Skin cancer has nothing to do with where you live.

14. Fair skin ages more quickly and runs a greater risk of developing skin cancer.

15. Strenuous exercise is harmful to your skin

16. Wrinkles, laugh lines, age spots and even freckles, can be removed by a chemical or non-surgical process.

17. After a chemical or laser facial rejuvenation, one may never go back out into the sun.

18. Children should be protected from excess sun exposure.

19. A cloudy day is unlikely to cause a sunburn or skin damage.

20. Sitting at a beach is more likely to cause a sunburn than being in your back yard.

21. Swimming at a pool, lake or ocean is more likely to cause sunburn than being in your back yard.

22. One can control the amount of tanning and prevent burning by choosing a specific sunscreen product.

23. It is possible to prevent any of the harmful sun's rays from reaching your skin.

24. Using an umbrella is guaranteed protection against sunburn.

ANSWERS

1. False	6. True	11. True	16. True	21. True
2. True	7. True	12. True	17. False	22. True
3. False	8. True	13. False	18. True	23. True
4. True	9. True	14. True	19. False	24. True
5. True	10. True	15. False	20. True	

Jean Osder, MD, of the Dermatology Associates Medical Group of Beverly Hills, reviewed the section on Skin Care Treatments.

Growing old is like being increasingly penalized for a crime you haven't comitted.

-Anthony Powell

APPENDIX B

A Summary Of Common Surgery Procedures At A Glance*

FACE AND NECK PROCEDURES

Common Term	Technical Term	Description of Procedure	Operating Room Time	Life of Operation	Stitch Removal Complete by	Return to Work or School by
Face and Necklift	Cervicofacial Rhytidectomy or Cervicalfacial Rhytidoplasty	Excess skin is removed from face and neck. Underlying muscles tightened. Excess fat is removed.	3 - 4 hours	10 -15 years	10 days	14 days
Nose Surgery	Rhinoplasty (Cosmetic)	Bone and cartilage are reconstructed and excess is removed from nose to reshape.	1-2 hours	Permanent	N/A**	7 days
	Septoplasty (Funtional)	Internal procedure to straighten the partition and improve airflow.	1 hour	Permanent	N/A**	7 days
Eyelid Surgery	Blepharoplasty	Elimination of fat and excess skin around the eye (removes bags and pouches).	1-2 hours	10 -20 years	5-7 days	7 days
Ear Surgery	Otoplasty	Cartilage of ears reshaped "pinning back" the ears.	1½ - 2 hours	Permanent	N/A**	7 days
Forehead/browlift	Browpexy	Lines and wrinkles modified through relaxing muscles, advancing tissue. Sometimes excess skin is removed.	1 - 2 hours	5 -10 years	10 days	10 -14 days
Chin Surgery	Mentoplasty	Implant to augement receding chin. Often performed with facelift or rhinoplasty to improve profile.	½ - ¾ hour	Permanent	5-7 days	5-7 days

* Modified from the *American Academy of Facial Plastic and Reconstructive Surgery* and the *American Society of Plastic Surgeons*

** N/A (not applicable) —Dissolving stitches used exclusively

FACE AND NECK PROCEDURES (continued)

Common Term	Technical Term	Description of Procedure	Operating Room Time	Life of Operation	Stitch Removal Complete by	Return to Work or School by
Double-Chin Surgery or Neck Sculpture	Submental Lipectomy	Fat deposits beneath the chin that result in the "double-chin" are removed or suctioned. Lax muscle may be tightened also.	1 hour	Usually permanent— if weight is stable	5 -7 days	7 days
Chemical Face Peel	Chemexfoliation or Chemical Facial Rejuvenation	Through a controlled burn with a caustic solution, the outer layer of skin is erased, giving the face a smoother texture. Performed to remove wrinkles, age lines and pigmentation irregularities.	1½ - 2 hours	Usually permanent	N/A	10 -14 days
Laser Face Peel		Destruction and resurfacing as in Chemical Peel but using a laser beam.	1½ - 2 hours	Uncertain, depends on type of laser	N/A	10 -14 days

BODY PROCEDURES

Common Term	Technical Term	Description of Procedure	Operating Room Time	Life of Operation	Stitch Removal Complete by	Return to Work or School by
Breast Augmentation	Augmentation Mammoplasty	Implant is placed to enlarge size or improve shape.	1½ - 2 hours	Permanent	7 -10 days	7 - 14 days
Breast Reduction	Reduction Mammoplasty	Large breasts are reduced in size and made firmer by the removal of excess tissue.	2½ - 3 hours	Permanent	7 - 21 days	10 - 21 days
Breast Lift	Mastopexy	The nipple is moved up and breast skin is brought down for support.	1½ - 2 hours	Permanent	7 - 14 days	7 - 14 days
Liposuction	Suction-Assisted Lipectomy	Fat suctioned from the thighs, hips, adomen, knees, face and under the chin.	¾ - 1 hour	Permanent	5 -10 days	5 - 14 days
Tummy Tuck	Abdominoplasty	Loose skin is is removed. Muscle tightening may also be performed.	2½ - 3 hours	Permanent	5 - 21 days	10 - 21 days

The goal of life is to die young - as late as possible.
-Ashley Montague

APPENDIX C
Recommended Reading Including Some Classics

The Smart Woman's Guide To Plastic Surgery, by Jean M. Loftus, MD, Contemporary Books, 2000. Excellent Resource. Unusually comprehensive, yet easy to read. Dr. Loftus delves into operative technicalities clearly illustrated with line drawings. The chapter explaining current treatments for skin discoloration, spider veins, tattoos, unwanted hair, stretch marks and cellulite is particularly strong. This book is highly recommended.

A Facelift Is A Bargain, by Nola Rocco, Hidden Garden Press, Beverly Hills, 1993. Nola operated one of Beverly Hills' original recovery hideaways. Her book includes The Beverly Hills Facelift Diet and The Hidden Garden Cookbook. In addition, Nola includes her "countdown to surgery": advice/instructions for sixty days, thirty, fifteen, ten, three, two and one day prior to surgery. Also, exactly what to wear and not to wear to your surgery appointment. A light, easy-reading book with some clever cartoons and warm patient commentaries. Worth your perusal.

Lift: Wanting, Fearing, and Having a Face-Lift, by Joan Kron, Viking, 1998. If you are limited to just one more book about cosmetic surgery (after completing this one, of course), this is the read. Joan Kron is the grand dame of writers who "cover" cosmetic surgery including its scuttlebutt, personalities and newer procedures. As an Editor at Large for *Allure* and author of its bimonthly feature, "Scalpel News," Joan is now regarded as the most savvy of the savvy, the capo de capo. She is a true superspecialist who must have a very strong antenna atop her New York co-op. She is always on top of "the latest" news and knows all the gossip and tidbits about the players in our rather unique specialty. Joan always gets it right. She checks, rechecks and double checks her facts through a huge network of informants and consultants. She even subscribes to cosmetic surgery medical journals!

When writing her book, Joan called me to ask some questions concerning the history of layman-performed, "underground" chemical skin peels. I was amazed at the digging she had done. My textbook *Chemical Rejuvenation of the Face* (Mosby Year-Book, 1991) included a well-sleuthed chapter on the history of chemical peeling. It was written by well-known medical historian Willard Marmelzat, MD of Tulane University Medical School. As comprehensive as was Dr. Marmelzat's historical review, Joan uncovered additional juicy tidbits. I swear she employs a cadre of former KGB agents; she is as "up" on the latest cosmetic-surgery-world gossip as she is on our specialty's "cutting edge" (pardon the pun) procedures. The book explores some of the deeper psychological dilemmas, hesitations and uncertainties with which anyone considering facial cosmetic surgery could identify. I highly recommend the book; it is a face lift encyclopedia.

Look Younger, Live Longer, by Gaylord Hauser. Fawcett Publications, Inc., Greenwich, Connecticut, 1951. This book has been in my library for a long time (It was published when I was nine years old!). Amazingly, the message is very contemporary. Hauser was one of the first diet and health specialists. His recommendations for healthy living have been quite accepted, although he was viewed originally as somewhat of a heretic. Very interesting reading.

Rejuvenate: Looking Younger And Feeling Vital, by Devra Z. Hill. Avery Publishing. Garden City Park, New York, 1991. Dr. Devra Hill is a unique woman. Depleted by her own illness years ago, and with no success from mainstream medicine, she became a student of alternative health options and an expert in nutrition and lifestyle. She has a list of clients that reads like Hollywood's Who's Who. Devra's new book is entitled, *The Best of Your Life—For the Rest of Your Life*. The book speaks of her natural, holistic approach to health and how the stars she's worked with have been able to look younger, feel better, and maintain high levels of energy without drugs or surgery The Hill genes must be very effective since Devra's twin daughters are coauthors of two natural foods cookbooks. The latest, a vegetarian cookbook, is entitled *Double Your Energy With Half the Effort.*

The End Of Aging: How Medical Science Is Changing Our Concept Of Old Age by Carol Orlock. Birch Lane Press. Secaucus, New Jersey, 1995. Carol Orlock is a writer who specializes in science and medicine. She presents a very easy-to-understand explanation of the aging process and why some of us look older than others. The book has some very interesting facts and concepts. Orlock notes that "around Julius Caesar's day, a half century before the birth of Christ, the average life expectancy in Rome was a mere 22 years. Fewer than 3 percent of men reached the age of 80; fewer than one percent of women." We have come a long way, indeed.

Redefining Beauty: Discovering Your Individual, Enhancing Your Self-Esteem, by Victoria Jackson with Paddy Calistro. Warner Books, New York, 1993. You have probably seen Victoria on her television infomercials which are very well done. The book demonstrates make-up techniques for different types of faces and shows you how to use make-up to maximize your features. Jackson's coauthor is Paddy Calistro, former beauty columnist for the *Los Angeles Times Magazine.* She has covered the arts, fashion and style for many local and national publications.

Age Erasers For Men: *Hundreds Of Fast And Easy Ways To Beat The Years,* by Doug Dollemore, Mark Giuliucci, and the editors of *Men's Health Magazine.* Rodale Press, Emmaus, Pennsylvania, 1994. This book covers a wide gamut of techniques, strategies, and advice for staying young, fit, and healthy. I was honored by being asked to write a section on cosmetic surgery.

Age Erasers For Women: Actions You Can Take Right Now To Look Younger And Feel Great, by the editors of *Prevention Magazine* Health Books, and the Rodale Center for Women's Health. Rodale Press, Emmaus, Pennsylvania, 1994. This book is the female analog to *Age Erasers For Men.* It covers the same spectrum and is equally well done. This book also includes a contribution from yours truly on cosmetic surgery of the neck. Rodale Press, publishers of *Prevention Magazine,* is one of the major (and best of the) health care publishers. Their focus is very sharp. What Rodale does is done well.

Psycho-Cybernetics: A New Way To Get More Out Of Life, by Maxwell Maltz, MD, FICS. Wilshire Book Company, 1960. Dr. Maltz was a respected plastic surgeon who recognized the power of improving one's "self image." The book was written in 1960, long before popularization of today's self-help gurus with their books and programs. His linkage of cosmetic surgery to one's positive self-image was a landmark observation.

Fast Face & Body Facts

- People between the ages of 35 and 50 made up 44 percent of those who had cosmetic plastic surgery in 2000 with more than 3.2 million procedures performed.

- People between the ages of 51 and 64 comprised 25 percent of all those having cosmetic plastic surgery last year with 1.8 million performed. The top three invasive surgical procedures for this age range were: eyelid surgery (154,969), face lift (75,846) and liposuction (70,838).

- The 19- to 34-year-olds compromised 20 percent of the total cosmetic surgery population with 1.4 million procedures performed. The top three invasive surgical procedures in this age range were: nose reshaping (141,955), breast augmentation (117,932) and liposuction (97,954).

- Cosmetic patients having multiple procedures at the same time is 26 percent.

-The 2001 Report of the 2000 Procedural Statistics,
American Society of Plastic Surgeons

Keep a watch also on the faults of the patients, which often make them lie about the taking of things prescribed.
                                        -Hippocrates (460-370 BC)

APPENDIX D
List Of Medicines And Herbs To Avoid Before Surgery

Aspirin And Aspirin-Like Products[*]

The following is a list of some of the most common aspirin products and nonsteroidal anti-inflammatory medications to be avoided two weeks prior to surgery and after surgery. It is by no means a complete listing. Therefore, you should be reading the labels of all medications you are taking—prescription or non-prescription.

Medicines to Avoid Before Surgery

4-Way Cold Tablets	Anacin Analgesic Arthritis Pain Formula	Axotal
A.P.C.	Anacin Analgesic Caplets and Tablets	Bac #3
Absorbent Rub	Anacin Maximum Strength	Bac Tablets
Absorbine	Analbalm	Banalg
Absorbine Jr.	Analgesic Balm	Bayer Aspirin — All Varieties
Act-On Rub	Antiphiogistine	BC Powders
Advil	Arthralgen	Ben-Gay
Alka-Seltzer Effervescent Antacid and Pain Reliever	Arthritic	Braska
Alka-Seltzer Extra Strength	Ascodeen-30	Buff-a-Comp
Alka-Seltzer Flavored Effervescent Antacids and Pain Reliever	Ascriptin with Codeine Tablets	Buffadyne
Alpha Phed Capsule	Aspercreme	Bufferin — All Varieties

[*] From John Williams, MD in *A Facelift is a Bargain* by Nola Rocco and Mickey Fine Pharmacy Staff, Beverly Hills, CA

Medicines to Avoid Before Surgery (Contined)		
Butalbital	Fiogesic Tablets and Capsules	Percodan Demi Tablets
Cama-Inlay Tabs	Glepirin Tablets	Persistin
Carisoprodol Compound	Heet	Rid-A-Pain
Celebrex	Ibuprofen (Motrin, Nuprin, Advil, Anaprox)	Robaxisal
Cheracol Liquid	Icy Hot	Roxiprin
Clinoril	Indocin	Rumarub
Congespirin	Infra-Rub	Sine-Aid
Cope	Lini-Balm	Sine-Off
Coricidin	Lodine	SK-65 Compound Capsules
Counterpain Rub	Lortab ASA	Sloan's
Damason-P	Measurin	Soltice
Darvon with ASA	Mentholatum	Soma Compound with or without Codeine
Darvon-N with ASA	Meprobamate and Aspirin Tablets	SPD
Dencorub	Midol	Stendin
DIET PILLS *	Monacet with Codeine	Stimurub
Di-Gesic Improved	Musterole	Supac
Doan's Rub	Naprosyn	Surin
Dolprin #3	Neurabaim	Synalgos DC Capsules
Duragesic	Norgesic	Talwin
Easprin	Norgesic Forte	Tolectin
Ecotrin	Oil-O-Sol	Triaminicin
Empirin with Codeine	Omega Oil	Vanquish
Emprazil	Orphengesic	Vioxx
End-Ake	Oruval	Vitamin E
Equagesic Tablets	Oxycodone	Voltaren
Esotrin	Pabirin Buffered Tablets	Yager's Liniment
Excedrin Extra Strength	Panalgesic	Zemo Liquid
Exocaine	Pepto-Bismol	Zemo Ointment
Feldene	Percodan	Zomax

* Prescription and nonprescription diet pills

ATTENTION!
Herbal Preparations Are Still Drugs. If You Are Taking Them, Do Not Keep Them A Secret.

Herbal medicinals or botanicals are increasingly popular. In 2001, Americans purchased more than $5 billion worth of these products.

While medical doctors do not necessarily object to their patients ingesting these nonprescription products, patients undergoing surgery are advised that:

> *There have not been enough studies of botanicals in the U.S. for us to state that there definitely will or will not be a reaction during surgery, but most anesthesiologists and surgeons will err on the side of caution...we do recommend discontinuing some herbal medications at least two to three weeks prior to surgery.* *

What particularly concerns me and other surgeons is that patients taking these substances often do not regard them as medicines. When asked, "What medications are you taking?" patients frequently do not reveal that they are taking these products. According to the American Society of Anesthesiologists, "Seven out of ten people using these will not tell their physicians." Our practice's unswerving routine is to raise the subject with all patients, at the "preoperative visit," several weeks prior to the surgery date. We give them the following list of the more common herbal medications and their potential complications that could arise during surgery:*

- **Ginseng** is used to enhance energy levels. If combined with stimulants, used by anesthesiologists, it can cause tachycardia and high blood pressure. It can also decrease the effect of warfarin, causing the blood to thicken and develop clots.

- **Ephedra** is included in over-the-counter diet aids. It interacts with inhalants used for anesthesia to affect blood pressure. If used with monoamine oxidase inhibitors or oxytocin, the patient can experience high blood pressure and irregular heart rate during surgery.

- **Feverfew** is often used to treat migraines. It inhibits platelet activity that can increase bleeding during surgery.

* Jessie A. Leak, MD, Associate Professor, Department of Anesthesia, MD Anderson Cancer Center, Houston. Dr. Leak is a researcher who specializes in the study of herbal medication.

- **Garlic** is used to lower lipids and as an antioxidant. It inhibits platelet activity, especially if the patient is already taking warfarin.

- **Valerian** is a mild sedative promoting sleep. It causes a potential increase in the effect of barbiturates used in anesthesia, creating a deeper effect from the anesthesia.

- **Ginkgo Biloba** is a circulatory stimulant. It decreases platelet activity and clotting ability.

- **St. John's Wort** is used to treat anxiety and depression. It may prolong the effects of some narcotics and anesthetics.

- **Licorice** treats symptoms of gastritis and duodenal ulcers. It can cause edema and chronic liver problems and increase the risk of renal insufficiency.

- **Echinacea** is used to enhance the immune system. It may cause hepatotoxicity and cause liver damage.

- **Ginger** treats nausea. It can increase bleeding time.

- **Goldenseal** is a diuretic and laxative. It can worsen edema and increase blood pressure.

COSMETIC SURGERY, IS STILL SURGERY. You've heard me say this previously and, hopefully, it is now ingrained in your "computer memory." We approach cosmetic surgery with the same care and concern that our neurosurgical colleagues do for brain surgery. Everything we do is important. For our patients, the procedure itself is not serious, but every precaution and safety element must be activated to reduce to near-zero the chance of any complication from surgery or anesthesia. But, remember, we need your help and cooperation.

> The most prevelent problema that we face as cosmetic surgeons are the interactions with the herbal medications and our patients' clotting systems. There are a number of herbal medications that increase the risk pf bleeding. One of the easy ways to remember a few of them is just memorize the gas, garlic, ginko (Asian), ginseng and giner. Those are allmedicines that will increase bleeding times and potentially cause difficulty for our patients.
>
> **Edmund Pribitkin, MD**
> in *Cosmetic Surgery Times*
> **September 2000**

CONSIDERING COSMETIC SURGERY?

A Handy 29-Point Checklist To "Check Out" Prospective Doctors And Their Surgical Facilities

Take A Copy To Each Consultation

Question	Yes	No	Notes
1. Is the majority of the doctor's practice devoted to cosmetic surgery?			
2. What percentage of the doctor's practice is cosmetic versus reconstructive plastic surgery?			
3. How long has the doctor been performing the procedure you are considering?			
4. How many of these procedures has he performed?			
5. Did the doctor learn to perform this procedure as part of his formal residency training or did he learn it after he completed his residency when he was in practice?			
6. Is the doctor board certified? Which board or boards?			
7. Has the doctor completed a full-time, six-month to one-year cosmetic surgery fellowship?			
8. Is the doctor a Fellow of the American College of Surgeons?			
9. Is the doctor or has the doctor been a medical school faculty member?			
10. Is the doctor a member of local, state and national medical societies? Which ones?			
11. Has the doctor written books or authored journal articles on the cosmetic surgery procedure(s) you are considering?			
12. Does the doctor teach other doctors his techniques of cosmetic surgery?			
13. How many of these procedures does the doctor perform in an average week?			

Questions (continued)	Yes	No	Notes
14. Does the doctor have hospital privileges to perform the procedure you are considering?			
15. Does the doctor have hospital admitting privileges in case of emergency?			
16. Is the surgery performed entirely by your surgeon? Or is part delegated to a surgeon-in-training?			
17. Will the doctor and the staff perform all postoperative care?			
18. Can you receive a copy of the doctor's professional biography which summarizes his training, qualifications and credentials?			
19. Where will the procedure be done? If in the doctor's office, has the operating room and recovery room been accredited by a recognized authority?; e.g., the Joint Commission on Accreditation of Health Care Organizations (JCAHO), The Accreditation Association for Ambulatory Health Care (AAAHC), or the American Association for Accreditation of Ambulatory Surgical Facilities (AAAASF)?			
20. If in an outpatient or ambulatory surgery center, is the center licensed by the state and/or certified by the U.S. Government? By JCAHO, AAAHC or AAAASF?			
21. Is the outpatient surgical facility located in a medical building?			
22. Will the anesthetic be administered by an anesthesiologist (physician specialist), nurse anesthetist or the surgeon?			
23. Is a recovery "hideaway" and transportation to and from the office available?			
24. Are typical "before and after" photos made available for your viewing? Do the results look nautral? Is the improvement significant?			
25. Does the office provide "computer imaging" to help you visualize the anticipated results of your procedure(s)?			
26. Can you speak and/or meet with a patient who has had surgery performed by the doctor?			
27. Does the office provide, at the consultation, an itemized "fee quotation sheet" listing all proposed services and charges?			
28. Does the office offer a financing program?			
29. What is the policy regarding charges for touch-up surgery?			

To all the innovative plastic surgeons of tomorrow: Hurry!!!
- Joan Rivers, author, *Don't Count the Candles*

Afterword
Even More Help For You

I want this book to help you be the smartest of consumers. It is my fervent desire to aid in your research and help direct you to a comfortable experience and superior result. This accomplished, you will derive satisfaction and years of pleasure.

Visit a Terrific Website

To help you further, may I suggest you visit our website: **www.robertkotlermd.com** We have built a site that is simple to navigate and packed with information. You can always learn more. Here are some of the unique features of the site:

- An 86 page online encyclopedia of cosmetic surgery.

- *About Face,* a 28-minute video featuring the experiences of seven male and female patients, plus segments from *Oprah* and other TV programs.

- 44 "before and after" photos.

- Highlights of key newspaper and magazine articles on cosmetic surgery.

- An online financing application.

- Links to other important sites.

- Computer imaging system—now, cosmetic surgeons can show you your "after"—if you mail or email your "before." All from the privacy of your home.

- Questions? We'll answer them.

- We're here to help, so feel free to contact us.

I'm anxious to hear from you. Let me know if this book helped you demystify the process of selecting a cosmetic surgeon.

436 North Bedford Drive, Suite 201
Beverly Hills, CA, 90210-4312
Telephone: (310) 278-8721, 9 – 5, PST,
Monday through Thursday
Fax: (310) 278-0114
My personal e-mail: rkotler@<u>robertkotlermd.com</u>

Performing cosmetic facial surgery for over 25 years has been a privilege. It has been an honor to have been chosen by thousands of patients to be the doctor who would make a profound and positive change in their lives. It is good work.

The responsibility is a heavy one, but the satisfaction is enormous. I have never had a boring day nor one in which I thought of doing other work. It has been a great run and I anticipate the future pleasure of helping many more achieve their desires. I say "Amen" to the following quotation:

> *"To love what you do and feel*
> *it matters, how could anything*
> *be more fun?*
> -Katharine Graham, former publisher ,
> *Washington Post*

Robert Kotler, MD, FACS
Beverly Hills, CA

INDEX

QUICK ORDER FORM

Give this book to a friend, loved one or colleague!

Internet Order: www.surgerysecrets.com
Telephone Order: 800-247-6553
Fax Order: 419-281-6883 (fax this form)
By Mail: Ernest Mitchell Publishers
           30 Amberwood Pkwy.
           Ashland, OH 44805

This book is also available at special quantity discounts for bulk purchases for sales promotions, premiums, fundraising or educational use. Please contact Ernest Mitchell Publishers at 888-599-3400.

☐ Yes, I want____copies of *Secrets of A Beverly Hills Cosmetic Surgeon* at $24.95 each plus $4.00 shipping and handling per book*. (Allow 15 days delivery.)

NAME_____

ORGANIZATION_____

ADDRESS_____

CITY_____STATE_____ZIP_____

EMAIL_____

* California address please add $2.00 for sales tax.

Payment (Please check one):

☐ Check or money order for:_____(check payable to Ernest Mitchell Publishers)

☐ Credit Card: ☐ Visa   ☐ MasterCard ☐ AmEx ☐ Discover

Card Number:_____

Name on Card: _____Exp.Date _____

Signature_____

www.surgerysecrets.com